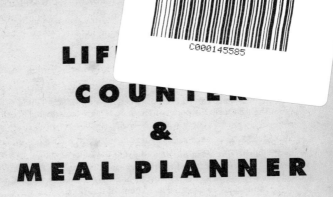

LIF
COUNTER
&
MEAL PLANNER

—

Peter Cox & Peggy Brusseau

THE ULTIMATE GUIDE TO THE WORLD'S
MOST POWERFUL FOOD CONTROL SYSTEM!

BLOOMSBURY

Publisher's Note

LifePoints is a registered trade mark of The Alta Vista Corporation Ltd protected by international copyright, trademark and service mark legislation. Unauthorized use is strictly forbidden. Manufacturers seeking permission to carry LifePoints labelling on products should apply to The Alta Vista Corporation Ltd at B. M. Box Superliving!,® London WC1N 3XX.

The information in this book was correct to the best of the Editor's and Publisher's belief at the time of going to press. While no responsibility can be accepted for errors and omissions, the Editor and Publisher would welcome corrections and suggestions for material to include in subsequent editions of this book.

This book may include words, brand names and other descriptions of products which are or are asserted to be proprietary names or trademarks. No judgement concerning the legal status of such words is made or implied thereby. Their inclusion does not imply that they have acquired for legal purposes a non-proprietary or general significance nor any other judgement concerning their legal status.

Please note that food products frequently change in composition, and this may substantially affect the ratings herein. A free update to the information in this book can be obtained from the address above. Please enclose a stamped addressed envelope.

This edition first published in 1997 by
Bloomsbury Publishing plc
38 Soho Square
London W1V 5DF

Copyright © 1997 The Alta Vista Corporation Ltd

The moral right of the authors has been asserted

A copy of the CIP entry for this book
is available from the British Library

ISBN 0 7475 3006 8

Typeset by Hewer Text Composition Services, Edinburgh
Printed and bound in Great Britain by
Cox & Wyman Ltd, Reading

AN IMPORTANT NOTE TO OUR READERS

All diets should begin with a medical check-up to make certain that no special health problems exist and to confirm that there are no medical reasons why you should not undertake a change of diet. Because the diagnosis and treatment of medical conditions is a responsibility shared between you and your medical advisors, neither the authors nor publisher of this book can accept responsibility for the individual consequences of dietary treatment based on the recommendations described herein.

The LifePoints system as described in this book has been created to be used by healthy adults. It does not apply to pregnant or lactating women, or to children. Women who are pregnant or lactating should not consider any weight-reduction diet until they have returned to a non-pregnant, non-lactating condition. A reduction in protein intake is emphatically not recommended for a woman who is pregnant or lactating as the health of her child relies on both a higher-protein and higher-calorie intake during this time.

LifePoints calculations for certain foods in this book have been based upon nutritional data published in McCance & Widdowson's *The Composition of Foods*. Data from *The Composition of Foods* has been used with the permission of The Royal Society of Chemistry and the Controller of Her Majesty's Stationery Office.

CONTENTS

JUST DO IT!

___

At this very moment, you have in your hands the world's most powerful and most versatile food control system. Not a fad diet, not a nine-day wonder . . . simply the most effective system ever created to give you what you really want from your food.

We spent many years creating the LifePoints system, because we wanted to use it ourselves. Probably like you, we were fed up with the quality of diet books on offer – many of them full of deceptive promises, most of them hopelessly impractical, and all of them forcing you to eat the kind of food that maybe suited the books' authors but sure didn't satisfy us!

There had to be a better way. We started by asking ourselves what we really wanted from our food – and we came up with three important answers.

Number one: weight control. As you'll almost certainly know from personal experience, most diet books can't even deliver this (*any* diet will work for a few weeks – virtually *none of them* work for longer). Most diet books make big promises, but they don't deliver – they should be put into the 'fiction' category in bookstores. As we've shown in *LifePoints Diet*, LifePoints can help you to lose weight and keep it off. So what if it isn't the fastest weight loss in the world? It's easy, it's healthy, and it lasts! 'I have been using LifePoints for 13 months', a reader recently wrote to us, 'in an effort to lose weight and have a healthier lifestyle. I have lost 35 lbs. As I am disabled my weight and general health are extremely important. I am delighted with the results and will continue using the books.' That's real, lasting success. Most diet books, however, assume that you're trying to win a medal in the dieting Olympics. What you end up being is a yo-yo.

Number two: supreme natural nutrition. Look at it like this: every day, you have a food 'budget' to invest. If you want to, you can fritter it away, consuming food which gives you absolutely no nutritional return on your investment. Or, you can choose food which will deliver a concentrated package of vital life-protecting nutrients, adding years to your life and life to your years. It's staggering – and shocking – to realize that until LifePoints there was no simple system like this to help you differentiate between foods.

Number three: fun! Somewhere along the way, haven't we all forgotten that food is really all about pleasure? What's the point in eating the healthiest diet in the world if it tastes like sawdust? If you've ever tried to follow a calorie-counting diet (and you need the brains of Einstein and a will of iron to do so) you'll know just how *guilty* food can make you feel. No one wants to be a slave to their diet, and, again, that's where LifePoints scores over all other regimes and diet books. LifePoints is as individual as you are – no matter who you are, or what your food tastes may be, LifePoints can perform superbly for you – guiding, encouraging, monitoring and assisting you so that you can achieve exactly what you truly want and really need from your daily food intake. LifePoints works for *you* – not the other way round.

But that's enough chat. You probably want to test-drive LifePoints right now . . . before another second has passed, without even reading this book. And the beauty of LifePoints is that you *can* put it to work for you in just a few seconds.

Try it now. Why don't you experiment with it for a few minutes, perhaps checking up on some of your favourite foods, and then – when you're ready – turn to Part One to learn more. Here's what you do:

1 Turn to the Counter (page 191) and browse through the list of thousands of foods until you find one or two which appeal.
2 Compare their LifePoints and RiskPoints numbers. LifePoints are a measure of a food's health-enhancing nutrients. Risk-Points are a measure of the food's less healthy ingredients. So you should aim to choose foods with a *high* LifePoints number, and a *low* RiskPoints number. With this simple but powerful insight, you can start to plan the healthiest diet you've ever eaten!
3 Your first priority is to ensure that you consume at least 100 LifePoints a day – more if you can! Isn't it nice to use a system which is *positive* about food – you'll quickly appreciate how LifePoints is a quantum leap beyond calorie counting. Choose foods as widely as possible from at least the first four groups. As far as RiskPoints are concerned, we suggest that your total daily intake shouldn't go above 100 or so.

Now you've learned just how simple the system is. It really does work the way you do – for example, if sitting down to plan your day's food intake doesn't temperamentally suit you, don't worry. Carry the book with you as you go through the day, and when you have to make a food decision, use it as your advisor. Should you go for the baked potato or the pasta? The Chinese meal or the Indian? In reality, all of us take lots of little food decisions like these all day long. And in the past there's been no way of deciding easily which is the best option. But with LifePoints to guide you, you can always make the right decision. And lots of little right decisions about your food intake add up to a major improvement in your diet! That's why we say: 'success by the inch is a cinch . . . by the yard, it's hard!'

No need to read any further for the moment . . . just do it!

Peter & Peggy
London

PART ONE: LIFEPOINTS GIVES YOU THE BIG PICTURE

———

If you've ever read a food label, you'll know what it is to be confused. All that data . . . yet so little information! 'Contains 45mg vitamin C per 100g', 'less than 1% of the RDI for calcium', '40g complex carbohydrate per 100g'. What language are they speaking? Martian? It's certainly not anything we earthlings can understand – or, more importantly, use.

Let's see. We have here, in front of us, a packet of healthy-looking crunchy oat cereal (well, oats are supposed to be good for us, aren't they?). Checking the 'Nutrition Information', we find that there are 9.6g of fat in every 50g of the cereal. Is that supposed to be good or bad? Some of that fat is saturated – 2.9g, to be precise – and 1.4g are polyunsaturated. Mmm. Then there are 5.4g of protein – now *that*'s supposed to be good for you, isn't it? And what else? Well, some 'energy' (we could all do with more of that!), lashings of carbohydrate, a dash of sodium and of course lots of healthy fibre. And that's all you learn from that – or any other – label. What happens if you put some milk on your crunchy oat cereal? It's been known to happen! It doesn't tell you. What happens if you eat more than the regulation 50g? And just how much is 50g in any case?

The nutritional 'information' on food labels has clearly been designed by an alien intelligence bent on world domination whose tactics are obvious – they're going to drive us all insane, and then take over the earth. It'll probably work, too.

And here's another example, which you must have seen many times: 'Contains 0.5mcg vitamin B12 per 100g. Average serving 28g.' That's *really* a wow. What you have to do (assuming you've got nothing else to do for the day) to find out how much vitamin B12 is in a serving is to divide 0.5mcg by 28 over 100. Are you still with us? Would you like your medication now?

Of course, it gets better still. Even if you perform all those mental gymnastics (and why would a nice person like you want to risk losing their mind?) you've still only calculated your intake of *one* nutrient, for *one* food, in *one* meal, for *one* day.

LifePoints takes the opposite point of view to all that insanity.

We say it doesn't really matter a fig whether there are 5g or 15g of fibre in your, er . . . fig. What counts is the big picture. Are you getting maximum nutritional value out of the food you're eating? Are you choosing the right foods to help you keep a trim weight? Where could you be doing better? That's what LifePoints is all about.

GOODBYE, CALORIE COUNTING – AND GOOD RIDDANCE!

When you think about food, you automatically think about calories. A fresh apple has about 80 calories. A tin of baked beans has about 300. A cheeseburger, about 600. And that's how we've been used to measuring the value of the food we eat – in terms of calories.

But calories are by no means a satisfactory gauge of a food's worth or importance to the human body and its wellbeing. What judgement can you truly make about a food which yields, say, 300 calories? Can you tell whether that food is good for you, or bad for you? Is it a healthy food or a health hazard? Will it tend to fortify or weaken your state of health? How well does it fit into the rest of your day's diet? Is it going to make you put on fat or lose weight? Does it contain health-enhancing nutrients, or disease-promoting antinutrients?

Calories can't begin to answer any of these vital questions. And yet, they are the only basis by which most of us have ever tried to assess the quality of the food we consume.

And what, in any case, is a 'calorie'? You may be surprised to find out. Calories have no tangible existence on their own – you can't see them, you can't taste them, and you certainly can't separate them out from the food itself. In Latin, 'calor' means 'heat', and that gives us a clue to the real rôle of the calorie. It is simply the name of a unit which we use to measure heat energy. One calorie was originally defined as the amount of heat energy required to raise the temperature of 1 gram of water from 14.5 °C to 15.5 °C. Pretty obscure, isn't it? Today, a calorie is defined in mechanical rather than thermal terms, so that 1 calorie equals 4.184 watt-seconds (or joules). Like feet, inches, metres, pints and litres, the calorie unit is a useful measure when used properly. For example, it takes 80 calories to melt 1 gram of ice. It takes 540 calories to boil 1 gram of water. Burn 1 gram of carbon and you'll release 7,830 calories. Run vigorously and you'll expend about 15,000 calories a minute (yes, we said '15,000'). Just to complicate matters, a 'calorie' when used in connection with food usually means a 'kilocalorie', or 1000 calories. Sometimes you'll see it written as 'kcal', and sometimes as 'Cal'. From now onwards in this book, we're going to follow the normal, although rather illogical, convention of saying 'calorie' when we really mean 'kilocalorie'. No one ever claimed that nutrition was a perfect science! This is all interesting enough, but what does it tell us about the quality of our food?

Nothing! Merely knowing the amount of heat energy locked up inside the food we eat isn't going to tell us much about that food's quality – or its impact on our health. Scientists tradition-ally used something called a 'bomb calorimeter' to measure the calorie yield of a food. They take a portion of the food in question – say a slice of cheesecake – and seal it inside a container. The air is pumped out, and oxygen gas is pumped in. Then, an electric spark ignites the oxygen and – bang! – the food burns and heat energy is released. The container is immersed in a water bath, and by measuring the rise in the water's temperature it is possible to calculate the calorie yield of the food. It doesn't sound much like your digestive system, does it?

So here we are, looking at food labels in the supermarket. We've already decided that trying to assess the nutrients given on a food label is a very quick route to the funny farm, so maybe reading the calories might help us?

Don't count on it (or them!). You've got two cans in your hands, now – both labels show approximately the same calorie yield. So which one are you going to choose? With only calories to work with, you might as well flip a coin.

Take another scenario. Now you're getting really professional at this calorie-counting business and you've bought a calorie counter. You've decided to limit yourself to about 1600 calories a day. So you diligently plan your day's food intake, calculator in hand, pencil and rubber near by. And holy mackerel, is it hard work! Juggling all those portion sizes, searching for a food which you can just squeeze into the limit – and, let's face it, doing a bit of cheating, too. Finally, you've done it – 1600 calories, or thereabouts. But what have you really achieved? Have you assured yourself a good intake of all the essential life-saving nutrients your body desperately needs? No! Have you made sure that your day's food intake is healthily low in fat? No!

Have you even managed to plan a diet which is going to help you lose weight? Well, what do *you* think?

THE CALORIE CON

When you drastically reduce your calorie intake, your body not unreasonably thinks you're starving. As far as your poor old bod is concerned, dieting and starving to death are one and the same thing. Now, starving to death is *not* good for your body but, happily, your body already has an excellent survival strategy all lined up, ready to be implemented at the drop of a calorie. The first thing it does is to lower your metabolism in order to conserve energy. The longer your food intake continues to be below what it expects, the harder your body tries to preserve that precious energy locked up as fat. That's why the first week or so of any diet always produces an impressive result yet subsequent weeks achieve little, if anything. Your body's deep-rooted instincts are fighting you all the way. And sooner or later they'll win. As they said in *Jurassic Park*, you can't fight nature!

One particularly notorious way in which your instincts triumph over your willpower is through the binge impulse. Anyone who's ever attempted dieting will be familiar with it. You may know the scenario – your diet's lasted a few days, and so far it's gone well. Then, in one insane and unrestrained moment, you find yourself behaving like a great white shark in a crowded swimming pool. Eat! Eat! Eat! As you maniacally bolt down everything that could possibly have a calorie or two associated with it, you start to feel helpless and, yes, ashamed. How could you possibly be so weak? How could you have ruined all your hard work in a momentary feeding frenzy? This sort of negative self-talk can sometimes even lead to serious eating disorders such as bulimia. But take it easy on yourself for a moment. When you think about it, the binge impulse is – yet again – a very logical and successful feeding strategy. Your body thinks that there is a severe food shortage which is causing you to starve. Trying to protect you, your instincts become super-sensitive to any potential source of food – and of course in today's society there are unlimited sources of food available everywhere. Drop your guard for just one instant and the ancient survival instincts take over.

And isn't dieting hell? Try as much as you can to put a brave face on it, you know it's sheer bloody misery really. You have to put up with absurdly small portions of your favourite foods, which requires superhuman discipline (or perhaps an unhealthy streak of masochism!). Even worse, you feel hungry most of the time, which makes you a real miseryguts to your colleagues, friends and family. Ever wonder why dieters have to club together in those self-help groups? It's because nobody else wants to talk to them.

Calorie-restricted diets have even more serious drawbacks, too. Have you ever noticed:

- Bloating and distended stomach
- Constipation
- Depression
- Failure to produce collagen, the major protein of all connective tissues
- Feeling cold all the time
- Hair loss
- Headaches
- Lack of energy
- Loss of lean tissue
- Low blood pressure leading to dizziness
- Menstrual difficulties
- Sleep disruption
- Water retention
- Yeast infections.

All of these problems have been associated with dieting in the scientific literature. In fact, there are enough scientific studies around now for us to come to the certain conclusion that dieting, as it's usually practised, is ineffective in any long-term sense. In a 1986 Dutch study, men who experienced many stressful life events in a short period experienced a weight gain. That's not unusual – once again, it's our body's way of trying to protect us from harm. A year later, this weight gain had disappeared in almost all subgroups of these men. The exception was the subgroup that tried to lose weight by dieting; those who dieted had gained yet more weight! This study, reported in the *International Journal of Obesity*, makes no sense to those who believe that weight gain is a 'calorie problem' and that weight loss can therefore be accomplished simply by restricting calories. But when you see it in terms of a survival strategy, it makes perfect sense: those men had already been through a number of stressful life events, and the threat of starvation (i.e. dieting) seemed, to their bodies, to be just one more hazard. Their bodies actually responded splendidly by trying to conserve every last calorie.

Many scientific studies now confirm that, if you want to put on weight, a great way to do it is to go on a diet. Weight gain is particularly provoked by 'diet cycling' (continual diet/binge cycles), and it is such a well-accepted phenomenon that it is sometimes used in a clinical situation to help underweight patients to put on bulk. How, precisely, does this happen? It's probably connected to the production of an enzyme called lipoprotein lipase (LPL) which is responsible for storing body fat. When you start a diet, LPL levels initially drop, then remorselessly rise again – sometimes to 25 times the normal level.

If calorie-restricted diets worked effectively there would be few people in the Western world with an obesity problem. In their recent paper entitled 'Diet and Health: Implications for Reducing Chronic Disease Risk', the Committee on Diet and Health of the National Research Council pointed out that 'food intake has declined over the past decade when body weight and presumably fat stores have, on average, increased'. In other words, our growing fatness cannot be explained by the fact that we're eating more calories – because we're not! Other studies have confirmed that Westerners today take in fewer calories than we did at the beginning of the twentieth century, while the level of obesity has stubbornly climbed.

So what have we learned so far? Three vitally important points:

1   Merely knowing the heat yield of a foodstuff as measured in calories tells us next to nothing about its real nutritional worth to us.

2   Conventional calorie-restricted diets have an extremely poor track record of success, and often ultimately lead to weight gain.

3   Since calorie-restricted diets don't work, and since we're consuming fewer calories today than we used to but are

getting fatter, we can reach the conclusion that effective weight control must involve more than just counting calories.

As you'll see, the LifePoints approach towards effective weight control is very subtle; you might call it 'the art of dieting without dieting'. We don't believe that crash diets are effective in the long run, nor are they necessarily safe for you. Neither do we believe that strict calorie counting usually achieves any worthwhile change. Instead, the focus of the LifePoints system is to trust our bodies and instincts a little more, while providing a helping hand and a system for developing and reinforcing our instinctive wisdom about the goodness or badness of our food choices. The LifePoints system can help you to regularize your weight by consciously directing you towards eating good food and avoiding bad.

It's that simple, because that's how we were designed.

YES, THERE ARE GOOD AND BAD FOODS

Plain common sense tells most of us that some foods are indeed better for us than others. When the American Dietetic Association released the results of a recent public opinion survey into attitudes towards food, they found that three out of four people surveyed believed that there are 'good' and 'bad' foods. That finding must have vexed doctrinal dieticians everywhere, because for years the profession has been telling us precisely the opposite – that virtually any food can be part of a 'well-balanced' diet.

Well, *someone* out there must be happily eating that legendary 'well-balanced' diet, because we hear so much about it all the time. Someone out there must be eating all the burgers, all the French fries, all the ice cream, all the other high-fat products and all the other foods we are so regularly told are just fine for us 'when eaten as part of a balanced diet'. But so far, we've never met them. All we see is evidence of people eating bad foods, and becoming fat and ill. Conversely, we see scientific studies following the health of people who eat good foods – and they *stay* slim and healthy.

Think critically for a moment about the myth of the 'balanced diet', and you'll soon realize just how preposterous it is. Here's how the myth goes: no food can be considered to be 'good' or 'bad', because virtually any food can be consumed providing it is done in the context of a balanced diet. This means, for example, that burgers, fries and milkshakes are fine, providing they are 'balanced' by the consumption of other foods.

All right. But precisely what 'other foods'? That's never made clear. We can assume, however, that those mysterious 'other foods' contain the health-enhancing nutrients which burgers, fries and shakes singularly lack. We can also assume that those 'other foods' *don't* contain the fats and other antinutrients which burgers, fries and shakes most certainly do contain. In other words, those 'other foods' are *good* foods.

Furthermore, foods such as burgers, fries and shakes contain absolutely no nutrients which can't be obtained from other food sources. Indeed, there are plenty of other foods which contain such nutrients as are found in burgers, fries and shakes – and which additionally *don't* contain the unhealthy fats and other antinutrient factors. So burgers, fries and shakes make no uniquely valuable contribution towards our overall good nutritional status, but they *do* contribute several undesirable antinutrients which we could well do without. In our book, that's a pretty good definition of a *bad* food.

So stripped down to basics, what they're actually saying is: it's OK to eat bad foods, as long as you also eat good foods.

Don't swallow it!

Good Foods Make Good Diets!

Before LifePoints, there was no simple way easily to check the nutritional worth of the food you ate. Although the raw data for food composition and the computing power to attempt the task were certainly available, the biggest problem was simply the prevailing mindset, characterized by that endlessly repeated mantra 'there are no good foods or bad foods, only good diets and bad diets'. Obviously, if there weren't any good foods or bad foods, there was no point in trying to rate them as such.

We thought differently. Applying decades of human population studies, we sought to assemble a picture of the major healthy and unhealthy factors in the human diet. For example, the evidence is overwhelming that people who consume significant quantities of saturated fat have a high incidence of heart disease –

so saturated fat is clearly a major risk factor in our diets. On the other hand, people who eat foods that are high in the antioxidant beta-carotene have much less heart disease and fewer cancers – which indicates that beta-carotene is one of the important health-protectors. Many of these nutritional factors will already be familiar to you. However, *never before* have you had the opportunity to see how they all add up to make a healthy or unhealthy food. Now, you can!

What do LifePoints actually measure? People sometimes expect the system to be measured in calories or some other familiar unit and are puzzled when it isn't. Well, think about it like this. Instead of measuring just one nutrient, LifePoints measures lots of them. First, we calculate an overall nutritional profile for the food being analysed, in its most common serving size. Next, we use a proprietary computer algorithm to compare the nutritional profile of that food with its respective 'ideal' nutritional profile and see how it fits. A good fit earns lots of LifePoints, a bad one earns none. It is important to emphasize that we're not just adding up all the nutrients in the food. That would produce a misleading result, since foods which contain very large amounts of just one or two nutrients would come out far too favourably. A food which has a high LifePoints number provides you with *lots* of nutrients in *beneficial* amounts. And if that food is also low in RiskPoints, then it's a *good* food. Simple, isn't it? These two numbers – LifePoints and RiskPoints – instantly provide you with a dynamic and enlightening picture of any food you care to look up! Now let's describe the importance of the wonderful nutrients which the LifePoints system relies upon.

WHAT'S IN A LIFEPOINT?
● **Beta-carotene**   The plant form of vitamin A, beta-carotene functions as a powerful antioxidant and free-radical quencher in the human body. The evidence is overwhelming that beta-carotene is one of the most important nutritional factors in your armoury against ill health. Popularly, beta-carotene is sometimes known as a 'cancer killer'. Men who eat very little beta-carotene have been shown to be seven times more likely to contract lung cancer than men whose diets are rich in it. In women, beta-carotene seems to be able to thwart cervical cancer.

Further, epidemiological evidence indicates that it can also reduce the incidence of cancers of the larynx, bladder, oesophagus, stomach, colorectum and prostate gland.

Today, we hear a great deal about antioxidants and free radicals. In the popular media free radicals are often characterized as 'bad', but, as with so many things, this is only partly true. The 'free-radical theory' was first proposed as long ago as 1954 by Dr Denham Harman, latterly Professor of Medicine and Biochemistry at the University of Nebraska. He discovered that radiation caused accelerated aging and also created an excess of free radicals in body cells. What is a free radical? Simply, an atom or molecule with an unpaired electron. It is inherently unstable, as it continually searches for another molecule to which to attach itself. Gerontologist Alex Comfort wittily compared a free radical to a convention delegate away from his wife. He called it 'a highly reactive chemical agent that will combine with anything that's around'. Free radicals trigger a chain reaction that 'rusts' the body. Free radicals can damage cell membranes, proteins, carbohydrates and deoxyribonucleic acid (DNA), the genetic material of the cell and of life itself. Up to now, some 60 diseases have been associated with free-radical activity, including Alzheimer's, heart disease, arthritis, multiple sclerosis and cataracts. Even liver spots – areas of brown skin which appear on your hands and arms later in life – are connected to free-radical activity. Although the body naturally produces free radicals, other substances – such as cigarette smoke, radiation, air pollution, herbicides, artificial flavourings, chlorine, rancid fats, alcohol and heavy toxic metals – are also causes of free-radical formation.

Free radicals aren't, however, all bad. There is persuasive evidence that the basic chemicals of life first originated in the 'primeval soup' from a series of free-radical reactions triggered by ionizing radiation from the sun. This would explain why free-radical reactions are so pervasive in nature. They enable genetic mutations to occur, and so play a pivotal rôle in the process of evolution. And your body deliberately produces free radicals when it wants to kill invading organisms, as part of its immune and inflammatory responses! Obviously, your body needs a system to manage free radicals effectively and, in particular, there has to be an effective protective and scavenging system to ensure that they don't get out of control. And that's what antioxidants do. In recent years, scientists have begun to appreciate just how crucial antioxidants are to our health. LifePoints delivers you a diet which is *naturally* high in many of the most powerful antioxidants.

There's no doubt that one very important aspect of the aging process is the damage which free radicals inflict on the human body. It is when things get out of balance between free radicals (pro-oxidants) and antioxidants that problems begin. If you're low on antioxidants you're wide open to free-radical attack. In fact, many scientists now suspect that what we call 'aging' is simply the final result of many free-radical reactions going on continuously through our cells and tissues.[1] If that view is correct the aging process might be amenable to alleviation and what we today consider to be an inevitable process might, tomorrow, be considered to be a disease process – and treated accordingly. After the age of 28, the greatest single risk factor for disease and death is the aging process itself.[2] It is shocking to realize that if one day all the major causes of premature death were eliminated, the average human lifespan would still be only 85 years.[3] And the only way we're going to extend that is by tackling the aging process itself.

Several scientific studies have already shown that dietary antioxidants can increase lifespan.[4] There's also powerful evidence from human populations that those people who take in bountiful amounts of natural antioxidants suffer far less from many killers such as cancer and heart disease. In America, the Alliance for Aging Research (which is a non-profit public health organization) recently assembled a panel of leading medical researchers, nutritionists and consumer safety experts to examine antioxidants and aging. They reviewed over 200 clinical and epidemiologic studies conducted over the past two decades, and concluded that 'a diet rich in antioxidants including beta carotene and vitamins C and E, is effective in guarding against heart disease, cancer, cataracts and other conditions associated with ageing'.[5]

Beta-carotene is a very powerful natural antioxidant, found in plants. It is turned into vitamin A in the wall of the small intestine during digestion. Of the several hundred naturally occurring carotenoids, beta-carotene is the most widespread and the most active. Foods which contain beta-carotene can be consumed in plentiful amounts without fear of toxicity. Beta-carotene is also:

- Essential for good eyesight
- Vital for tissue growth and bone development
- Used to maintain the integrity of mucous membranes, thus building a barrier against infection
- Necessary for the proper growth and functioning of the reproductive system.

Sometimes people ask us why they can't just eat an indifferent diet and rely on vitamin supplements to make up any nutritional shortfall – as a kind of 'nutritional insurance policy'. Well, the case of beta-carotene illustrates why you shouldn't follow this route. Taking beta-carotene, and indeed all nutrients, in its natural form is extremely important. In nature, *nothing works in isolation*. This was dramatically underlined recently, when the results of a long-awaited major study came to the startling conclusion that high doses of beta-carotene, when taken in capsule form, can actually *raise* the risk of cancer rather than lower it!

The study was intended to show whether beta-carotene protects smokers from lung cancer. Instead, it found that those taking the isolated vitamin *increased* their lung cancer risk by 18 per cent. The ten-year, $43 million study was conducted on 29,133 male cigarette smokers who lived in Finland. Smokers were chosen because they are already at high risk of lung cancer and beta-carotene appeared to be an especially promising way to lower the chance of this disease.

Now don't misunderstand this study. It does *not* suggest that foods which naturally supply a plentiful amount of beta-carotene can increase your risk of cancer! Quite the opposite. Decades of studies tracking the health of thousands of people prove beyond doubt the wisdom of eating beta-carotene-rich foods. But as to whether it's wise to replace this sort of food with a pill – well, that's not such a good idea. Happily, you now have LifePoints to give you a way of assessing the broad nutritional profile of many different kinds of foods. It's a holistic approach – and the healthiest.

● **Vitamin C**   Although it was long considered as relevant only to the prevention of scurvy, there is now abundant evidence that a first-class intake of vitamin C can help to prevent a vast range of human diseases. Humans are one of the few species unable to synthesize vitamin C internally, and therefore we need to be certain of a regular, high-quality dietary intake. Vitamin C is also a very effective antioxidant and free-radical quencher. You can even see it at work for yourself. Cut an apple in half, and put one half aside. Pour lemon juice, which is high in vitamin C, on the other half. The half without the lemon juice will go brown through oxidation much faster than the half which is protected by the antioxidant vitamin C. In a recent study conducted at the University of California at Berkeley, scientists isolated plasma from human blood, incubated it at body temperature and added a chemical that is known to produce free radicals as it decomposes. When vitamin C was added it neutralized 100 per cent of the free radicals generated. Vitamin C also:

- Assists in the production of collagen, a protein which is the body's building block for all connective tissue, cartilage, bones, teeth, skin and tendons
- Helps wounds, fractures, bruises and haemorrhages heal
- Maintains the function of the immune system
- Greatly facilitates the absorption of iron
- Assists haemoglobin and red blood cell production
- Is an essential co-factor for metabolism of many other nutrients
- Helps the body cope with physiological and psychological stress.

Vitamin C also seems to block the formation of nitrosamines. Nitrates and nitrites are added to foods to give colour, flavour and to act as preservatives (E249–E252). During digestion these substances are converted by the human body into nitrosamines, which are known to be powerful cancer-causing chemicals (they are particularly associated with cancers of the stomach and the oesophagus). The good news is that if a vitamin-C-rich food is taken at the same time as foods containing nitrates or nitrites the production of nitrosamines is greatly reduced. It has also been found that women with abnormal cervical smear results often

13

have low amounts of vitamin C in their bodies. This may shed new light on the underlying damage caused by smoking, because it has long been established that women who smoke have higher levels of cervical cancer. Smoking impairs the absorption of vitamin C.

● **Thiamin**   Also called thiamine or vitamin B1, thiamin was discovered to be the nutritional factor responsible for preventing the disease beriberi (Sinhalese for 'I cannot', meaning that the sufferer is too ill to do anything). Epidemics of beriberi were caused in Asia by a diet of white polished rice, where all the nutritional content of the outer layers of rice is discarded during processing. Although beriberi is primarily a disease of tropical countries, nutritional deficiencies of thiamin are also seen in the West – especially amongst people who eat a typically highly refined, junk food diet. In the body, thiamin functions to:

● Convert carbohydrate into energy for the muscles and nervous system
● Keep mucous membranes healthy
● Maintain a positive mental state and, possibly, assist learning capacity.

● **Riboflavin**   Also known as vitamin B2, riboflavin was first observed in 1879 as a greenish fluorescent pigment present in milk, but its function was not fully understood until 1932. It is often found in combination with other B-group vitamins, and since it is not stored in the human body for any period of time it is vital that your diet supplies regular amounts. A deficiency will result in cracked and scaly skin; soreness of lips, mouth and tongue; and sometimes heightened sensitivity to light, watering of eyes or conjunctivitis. In the body, riboflavin works:

● With other vitamins and enzymes in the utilization of energy from food
● To keep mucous membranes healthy
● As a key component in normal tissue respiration.

● **Niacin**   Also called vitamin B3, niacin is the collective name for nicotinamide (niacinamide) and nicotinic acid. Its importance was realized in 1937 when it was discovered that the disease pellagra was caused by niacin deficiency. Lack of niacin in the diet can also lead to fatigue and muscle weakness, loss of appetite and mental unbalance. In the body, it plays an important rôle in:

- The release of energy from carbohydrates, fats and proteins
- DNA synthesis
- Keeping the skin, nerves and digestive system working healthily.

● **Vitamin B6** Also known as pyridoxine, vitamin B6 is (in common with other B-group vitamins) soluble in water. This means that the body's storage capacity for B6 is limited, and we need to ensure a good daily dietary intake. It works in the body to:

- Manufacture and convert amino acids and metabolize protein
- Produce haemoglobin
- Convert the amino acid tryptophan to niacin
- Facilitate the release of glycogen for energy from the liver and muscles
- Help the body process linoleic acid (an essential fatty acid)
- Help build and maintain the integrity of the nervous system and brain.

● **Vitamin B12** Also called cobalamin, this vitamin is manu-factured by micro-organisms such as yeasts, bacteria, moulds and some algae. The human body can store this vitamin for considerable periods (5 to 6 years) so a daily dietary source is not essential. In addition, the healthy body recycles this vitamin very effectively, recovering it from bile and other intestinal secretions, which is why the dietary requirement is so low (being measured in millionths of a gram). However, B12 deficiency is an occasional problem for people on restricted diets, and in view of its importance it is wise to consume a known B12 food source from time to time. Its functions in the body are to:

- Facilitate the normal metabolic function of all cells
- Work with folate to prevent anaemia

- Assist in the process of DNA synthesis
- Promote the growth and normal functioning of the nervous system.

- **Folate** Folate and folacin (sometimes called vitamin B9) are the names used to describe a group of substances which are chemically similar to folic acid. Folate's importance for growth and the prevention of anaemia was established in 1946. The name 'folate' comes from the Latin word *folium*, meaning a leaf, which should tell us something about the best sources of this vitamin. In the body, it:

- Plays an essential role in the formation of DNA and RNA
- Functions together with vitamin B12 in amino acid synthesis
- Is essential for the formation of red and white blood cells
- Contributes to the formation of haem, the iron constituent of haemoglobin.

- **Calcium** The most plentiful mineral in the human body, calcium makes up 1kg or so of the average adult's weight; 99 per cent of this is deposited in the bones and teeth, with the remainder fulfilling essential regulatory functions in the blood and cellular fluids. The body stores its skeletal calcium in two ways: in the non-exchangeable pool (calcium which is on 'long-term deposit' in the bones) and in the exchangeable pool, which can act as a short-term buffer to smooth over the peaks and troughs in day-to-day dietary calcium intake. If dietary intake is consistently too low then the exchangeable pool of calcium will become so depleted that the calcium on 'long-term deposit' in the bones will be put to use, thus inducing bone degeneration.

Although calcium is often thought of as the 'bone mineral', the 1 per cent of serum calcium in the human body (calcium held outside the skeletal structure) is responsible for a vital and complex range of tasks. Calcium is clearly a critical nutrient, and we all need to ensure that we have an intake of it. Many people erroneously believe that the consumption of heroic quantities of dairy produce is the only way to prevent bone-depleting afflictions such as osteoporosis. This is not so. The landmark 'China Study' (see page 20) showed that although the Chinese take in only half the amount of calcium that Westerners do, osteoporosis is rare in China. Why should this be? Well, most Chinese eat no dairy products and instead get all their calcium from vegetables. This is why we've included the calcium content of all foods in the LifePoints equation. We'd like you to get a good calcium intake from a wide variety of foods, rather than assuming that large amounts of milk and dairy products will protect you. In fact, studies among Western vegetarians and meat-eaters show that people who eat meat and dairy products are significantly more at risk of bone loss than non-meat eaters. Calcium also functions in the body to:

- Help build and maintain bones and teeth
- Help control the transportation of chemicals across cell membranes
- Facilitate the release of neurotransmitters at synapses
- Influence the function of protein hormones and enzymes
- Help regulate heartbeat and muscle tone
- Initiate blood clotting.

● **Iron**   We all know that iron prevents anaemia and is essential for haemoglobin production. As such, it is involved in the transportation of oxygen from the lungs to the body's tissues, it transports and stores oxygen in the muscles, and it is involved in the proper functioning of the immune system and intellect. Iron deficiency is the most common of all deficiency diseases in both developing and developed countries. Scientists vary in their estimate of what precisely constitutes a state of 'iron depletion', but the general cut-off point is variously calculated to lie between 12 and 25mcg of ferritin (one of the chief iron storage forms) per litre of plasma. In Britain, a recent survey showed that 34 per cent of all women had a ferritin level under 25 mcg/l, and 16 per cent had one under 13 mcg/l. Amongst men, only 6 per cent had a value of less than 25 mcg/l, and 3 per cent less than 13 mcg/l.

These figures reflect the fact that iron is conserved well by the body (90 per cent of the 3 to 5g in our bodies is continually recycled). The major cause of iron depletion is loss of blood itself – as in menstruation, which on average causes about 0.5 mg of iron to be lost for every day of the period. However, this can vary very widely (losses as high as 1.4mg per day have been reported), so the official recommended daily allowances for women attempt to take this into account by building in a generous safety margin. For example, an iron intake of 10.8mg per day appears to meet the needs of 86 per cent of all menstruating women,[6] yet the official American recommended daily allowance has been set at 15mg per day in an attempt to meet the needs of the remaining 14 per cent. This is, in fact, an uneasy compromise, because even at this level of iron consumption 5 per cent of women who have very heavy periods will not have an adequate intake to replace losses. At this point, the officials suggest either that women with higher blood losses appear to compensate with an increased rate of iron absorption from their diets (American) or that 'the most practical way of meeting their high iron requirements would be to take iron supplements' (British). This well illustrates the dilemma facing officials whose task it is to set uniform nutritional intakes for a population whose individual needs naturally vary very widely indeed. The rate of absorption of iron from the diet can be significantly affected, for better or worse, by several factors:

1   The rate of iron absorption is controlled by the degree to which iron is actually *needed* by the body. Normally, only 5 to 15 per cent of the iron in food is actually absorbed, but this can rise to 50 per cent in cases of iron deficiency.

2   Foods containing vitamin C will considerably increase iron absorption. Iron must be delivered in a soluble form to the small intestine if it is to be absorbed, and vitamin C can make sure that non-haem iron (the sort found in plant foods) remains soluble in the acidic environment normally found there. Other organic acids found in fruit and vegetables, such as malic acid and citric acid, are also thought to possess this iron-enhancing attribute. This effect is substantial: adding 60mg of vitamin C to a meal of rice has been shown to more than triple the absorption of iron; adding the same amount to a meal of corn enhances absorption fivefold. The LifePoints formula includes both iron and vitamin C.

3   The tannin in tea can significantly reduce the absorption of iron, by combining with it to form insoluble iron compounds. The food preservative EDTA can also exercise the

same inhibitory effect. Both of these factors can reduce assimilation by as much as 50 per cent.

● **Zinc** The human body contains a mere 2g of zinc, distributed in the tissues in varying concentrations. Its importance to good human nutrition has only been recognized in recent years (the first reports appeared in 1963). Low zinc status often manifests in a decrease in the senses of taste and smell, wounds take longer to heal and children fail to grow properly. This is because, in the human body, zinc is:

● An essential component of many enzymes which work with red blood cells to transport carbon dioxide from tissues to lungs
● A vital factor in many key life processes, such as our immune function and the expression of genetic information.

In addition to all the nutrients mentioned above, the LifePoints number also assesses foods for their fibre content (which, as you must know, imparts a whole host of health benefits, ranging from the prevention of various forms of cancer to lowering blood cholesterol and preventing constipation) and their protein content. *A high LifePoints number indicates that the food concerned is a beneficial source of nutrients. A low number indicates that it is a poor source.*

WHAT'S IN A RISKPOINT?

There is one huge risk factor in the diets most of us eat today, and that is the amount of fat consumed. Fat – and in particular saturated fat (mainly from animal sources) – is without doubt our number one dietary enemy. Most of us already know that eating too much fatty food is bad for us. But we'll bet you *didn't* know these shocking and startling facts:

● Eating 100 calories from fat will make you put on more weight than eating 100 calories from carbohydrate. On the face of it it seems impossible; after all, 100 calories is 100 calories . . . no matter where it comes from – right? Wrong! Your body stores surplus energy intake in the form of fat. When you eat fatty foods, your body can very easily and very efficiently turn that food fat into body fat. Only about 3 per cent of the fat you consume is burned up by your body in the storage process.[7] Building massive hips and thighs has never been easier! However, the process of turning carbohydrate-rich foods into body fat consumes a considerable proportion (about 25 per cent) of their calories. Further, carbohydrate-rich meals will themselves boost your body's metabolism, which in itself makes it harder for you to gain weight. Fatty foods simply don't have this effect.

- If you want to control your weight, all types of fat are equally bad. Forget the advertising slogans about polyunsaturates and monounsaturates; none of them help you shed those pounds. One gram of fat – of any kind – yields twice as many calories as a gram of protein or a gram of carbohydrate. *Fat is a poor nutritional return on your food investment.*

- A naturally low-fat diet can do remarkable things, including reverse heart disease. Scientifically, there's no doubt. The plaques which build up and eventually block coronary arteries can be unblocked by eating a healthy, low-fat diet. Amongst other benefits, increased flow of blood in these arteries can also reduce the pain of angina.[8]

Watching that RiskPoints number helps to ensure that your fat consumption remains healthily low. How low? Well, if your RiskPoints daily total adds up to no more than 100, you'll have eaten no more than 40 grams of fat. For the average woman, whose energy intake comes to about 2200 calories, that represents 16 per cent of calories. For a man, consuming about 2900 calories, it keeps your total fat intake down to about 12 per cent of calories. These are the kinds of levels which research shows our species has naturally consumed for most of its history. In many parts of the world – China, for example – people still consume this (to us) relatively low level of fat in their diets. The result? Many of the 'diseases of civilization' which so plague us in the West are virtually unknown. Why do we choose this level? Here's how the *New York Times* put it when reporting the results of the largest ever scientific study into the diets and health of the Chinese people: 'Reducing dietary fat to less than 30 per cent of calories, as is currently recommended for Americans, *may not be enough* to curb the risk of heart disease and cancer. To make a significant impact, the Chinese data imply, a maximum of 20 per cent of calories from fat – and preferably only 10 to 15 per cent – should be consumed.'[9] The 'China Study' is a turning point in the science of epidemiology. The study began in 1983, with the aim of exploring the dietary causes of cancer. Since then, it has been expanded to include heart, metabolic and infectious diseases. This seminal study has shown that obesity is clearly related to *what* you eat, rather than *how much*. The Chinese actually consume 20 per cent *more* calories than Westerners do, but Westerners are 25 per cent fatter! The culprit? All that fat in our food.

ARE YOU A FAT ADDICT?

Reducing fat consumption to 100 RiskPoints or so can be a challenge for some people. Fat is one of the most pervasive ingredients in today's food, and especially in fast food. You can quickly become addicted to a high-fat diet, to the extent that you'll search out high-fat foods in preference to more healthy offerings. You can check the degree to which you may be a 'fat addict' by doing the following quiz, devised by clever researchers at Seattle's Fred Hutchinson Cancer Research Center. Here's how to do it:

Think about your diet over the past three months and answer each of the questions by choosing a number from 1 to 4. If a question doesn't apply to your diet, leave it blank (for instance, if you don't eat red meat, don't answer questions 5, 6, and 19 – your score is based on the rest of your diet).

1 = Always
2 = Often
3 = Occasionally
4 = Rarely or Never

	In the past three months, when you . . .	Your answer 1 to 4
1	Ate fish, did you avoid frying it?	
2	Ate chicken, did you avoid frying it?	
3	Ate chicken, did you remove the skin?	
4	Ate spaghetti or noodles, did you eat it plain or with a meatless tomato sauce?	
5	Ate red meat, did you trim all the visible fat?	
6	Ate ground beef, did you choose extra lean?	
7	Ate bread, rolls or muffins, did you eat them without butter or margarine?	
8	Drank milk, was it skimmed milk instead of full fat?	
9	Ate cheese, was it a reduced-fat variety?	
10	Ate a frozen dessert, was it sorbet, ice milk or a non-fat yogurt or ice cream?	
11	Ate cooked vegetables, did you eat them without adding butter, margarine, salt pork or bacon fat?	
12	Ate cooked vegetables, did you avoid frying them?	
13	Ate potatoes, were they cooked by a method other than frying?	
14	Ate boiled or baked potatoes, did you eat them without butter, margarine or sour cream?	
15	Ate green salads with dressing, did you use a low-fat or non-fat dressing?	
16	Ate dessert, did you eat only fruit?	

17	Ate a snack, was it raw vegetables?	
18	Ate a snack, was it fresh fruit?	
19	Cooked red meat, did you trim all the fat before cooking?	
20	Used mayonnaise or a mayonnaise-type dressing, was it low-fat or non-fat?	

Now it's time to learn the truth! First, transfer the numbers above to the score sheet below. Disregard questions that were left blank. You'll see that the items are arranged within five fat-lowering strategies rather than according to their order in the quiz. Add up the total for each strategy, then whip out your calculator and follow the instructions . . .

Strategy 1: How well do you avoid frying your food?

Question 1 _____

Question 2 _____

Question 12 _____

Question 13 _____

Subtotal _____

Now divide by 4 to learn your average: _____

Strategy 2: How well do you avoid fatty meat?

Question 3 _____

Question 5 _____

Question 6 _____

Question 19 _____

Subtotal _____

Now divide by 4 to learn your average: _____

Strategy 3: How well do you avoid fat as a flavouring?

Question 4   _____

Question 7   _____

Question 11   _____

Question 14   _____

Subtotal   _____

Now divide by 4 to learn your average: _____

Strategy 4: How well do you substitute low-fat or non-fat versions of foods?

Question 8   _____

Question 9   _____

Question 10   _____

Question 15   _____

Question 20   _____

Subtotal   _____

Now divide by 5 to learn your average: _____

Strategy 5: How well do you replace fatty foods with fresh produce?

Question 16   _____

Question 17   _____

Question 18   _____

Subtotal   _____

Now divide by 3 to learn your average: _____

Now add up all your averages and write the grand total here: _____. Finally, divide this figure by 5 to calculate your overall score, and write it here: _____. Then check the chart below:

If your overall average is	Your percentage of fat from calories is	And we say
1 to 1.5	Under 25%	Excellent!
1.5 to 2	25 to 29%	Better than most people – a few small tweaks and you're there
2 to 2.5	30 to 34%	Some of your eating habits need attention, but there's hope!
2.5 to 3	35 to 39%	Most people's scoreline – you need a LifePoints makeover!
3 to 3.5	40 to 44%	Your diet's putting you at risk
3.5 to 4	45% or more	Fat addict level – LifePoints can help you, but you'll also have to retrain your tastebuds to enjoy less fatty food

Make sure you take the Fat Check again when you've completed your first month on LifePoints! You'll be pleased and encouraged by the progress you've made.

One of the nice things about the LifePoints system is that it's very forgiving. If you blow it completely one day – say for a party or some other kind of debauchery – it's no big deal. Just use the system to get yourself back into shape again over the next few days. Although we suggest a RiskPoints limit of about 100, you can adjust this to suit your own very individual requirements (another fact or that most other diets ignore). If you want to use the system for weight loss, here are some suggested RiskPoints limits:

RiskPoints limit	Potential for weight loss
75	Allows 30g of fat per day – the lowest suggested limit
100	Allows 40g of fat per day – maintains weight loss
125	Allows 50g of fat per day – gradual weight loss still occurs

Don't be dismayed if you check up the RiskPoints ratings for some of your favourite foods, and see that with one or two servings, you've exceeded your daily limit. Remember that there are plenty of foods whose RiskPoints ratings are extremely low – and with just a browse through the Counter, you'll quickly find them. In 'The LifePoints Makeover', we'll hold your hand as we walk through a number of real-life examples of tweaking and transforming diets to make them shine!

RISKPOINTS – BEYOND FAT COUNTING

Now, the RiskPoints number does a lot more than just keep track of the total amount of fat you've consumed. As you may know, many dieters have forsaken calorie counting in favour of fat counting – because counting the amount of fat in a food is easier to do and it produces better results. Well, the RiskPoints number is even better than fat counting. Here's why: the RiskPoints number intelligently guides you away from food which is unhealthily high in saturated fat, and steers you towards food which is low in it. Why is this important? Because saturated fat is clearly linked to the development of coronary heart disease and probably to certain cancers too. In this respect, all fat is *not* the same. We don't want you getting all your fat intake as unhealthy saturated fat. So the RiskPoints formula penalizes foods which are too high in this type of fat. You can think of this part of the RiskPoints equation as a silent friend there in the background, gently nudging you away from unhealthy foods and leading you to the healthier choices. One RiskPoints number serves two important functions. You may not notice it, but it's there, working for you all the time!

Now you can see why we say that LifePoints is 'beyond calories'. It really is the world's most advanced – and easiest – food control system. Imagine what would happen if all the world were to eat a natural diet which was high in LifePoints and low in RiskPoints. Actually, we don't have to imagine. The science of epidemiology already suggests what many of the benefits could be:

- Immune functioning enhanced
- Coronary heart disease defeated
- Incidence of many cancers reduced
- People's lives extended to an active older age, where they feel healthier
- Cataracts reduced
- Osteoporosis reduced
- High blood pressure prevented and treated
- Strokes reduced
- Impotence reduced
- Obesity prevented and treated
- Arthritis reduced
- Gout reduced
- Diabetes prevented and treated
- Hypoglycaemia prevented and treated
- Constipation prevented and treated
- Varicose veins prevented and treated
- Appendicitis prevented and treated
- Gallstones prevented and treated
- Food poisoning reduced.

Now you know the basics of the LifePoints system. The next thing is to get it working for you!

PART TWO: THE LIFEPOINTS MAKEOVER

The moment has arrived! It's time to put the past behind you, and discover a healthy new way of eating – and living. On this voyage of discovery, the LifePoints system will be your friend and guide.

Because people are so accustomed to diets which boss them around and tell them precisely what they may or may not eat, they sometimes find the freedom of the LifePoints system rather strange. To help you adjust to life outside 'diet prison', we've written this section of the book to gently hold your hand as we walk through the system in real life. You'll see just how easy it is radically to transform *any* diet into something that glows with health. First, let's make the principles of LifePoints absolutely clear.

THE THREE LIFEPOINTS LAWS

1 *Eat healthily*! Dieters are notoriously bad eaters – you know what we mean. Your first and prime objective is to score at least 100 LifePoints – more if you can.

2 *Eat for variety*! For your convenience, we have divided foods into six major groups. To eat a healthy and varied diet, you *must* choose foods from the first four groups. Groups 5 and 6 are optional. The suggested number of servings per day from each group is listed below:

Group 1	Fruit and Fruit Juices	3 servings
Group 2	Cereals, Grains and Pasta	4 servings
Group 3	Vegetables and Vegetable Products	4 servings
Group 4	Legumes, Nuts and Seeds	3 servings
Group 5	Meat, Fish and Dairy	optional
Group 6	Drinks, Desserts, Snacks and Sauces	optional

3 *Don't be boring!* We'll say it again – variety is the keynote of healthy eating. To encourage you to eat as wide a variety as possible, you must observe this rule: the LifePoints for any foodstuff can only be counted once, no matter how often you eat that food during the day. This means that if you eat the same food twice, only its RiskPoints count for the second helping. In other words, don't try to cheat the system by eating 10 servings of broccoli for 120 LifePoints and only 10 RiskPoints! (If you ever did eat ten helpings of broccoli, using this simple rule you'd accumulate 10 RiskPoints but only 12 LifePoints.) Foods are listed in common serving sizes, but it's quite acceptable to halve or even quarter the servings, providing you also reduce the associated RiskPoints and LifePoints.

THE LIFEPOINTS HIT LIST: SEARCH AND DESTROY

Once you have resolved to gain health and eat a healthier diet, you are ready to grasp the nettle and make the changes necessary to achieve your goals. Your first step must be to identify the weak spots in your diet – those aspects of your diet that one way or another deprive you of good health. But don't worry – you're not alone! In our experience, most people suffer from similar diet deficiencies, which we've shown below as 'targets' for you to identify and sort out. Here is the LifePoints Hit List: a five-target search and destroy mission that will culminate in a food 'holiday', a seven- to fourteen-day period of wholesome eating we have called the LifePoints Lift-Off.

Target One

Your diet is weak if it lacks *variety*. Keep a record of the food you eat for up to one week (use the Daily Food Planner on page 46). Include every food item and use the Counter to attribute LifePoints and RiskPoints to each food. Also, notice to which group each food belongs and tick the appropriate column. Total each column every day. Now compare the number of servings you ate from each food group to the number we suggest (see page 29). By the end of the week, you will have a pretty clear idea of what food groups you need to eat a little more from to ensure greater variety in your diet.

> Destroy! *Any overuse of Groups 5 and 6, especially at the expense of foods from the four essential food groups.*

Target Two

Your diet is weak if you have one or more meals that are always the same. For instance, many people eat the same breakfast day in and year out. This not only means lack of variety in your diet, but it also stops you from trying new foods that will help in developing an excellent diet. If this sounds like you, make a special effort to try a new and different menu for your stuck-in-a-rut meal. You will see plenty of ideas in the Meal and Menu Collections, later in the book.

Destroy! *Monotony, repetitiveness and stuck-in-tradition habits.*

Target Three

Your diet is weak if you overuse one or more foods. For instance, many people have a tea or coffee habit which means they consume milk, milk and more milk day after day. By the end of the day, the RiskPoints can really mount up from this one food alone, and that can prevent you from enjoying other more healthy foods. Many people also overuse bread, butter or even potato. Look through your Daily Food Planner to discover an overabundance of one food item. Now browse through the food listings to discover new and healthier options that will add variety and interest to your diet.

Destroy! *Mono-diets and bulk consumption of single food items.*

Target Four

Your diet is weak if you use too many double-zero foods. There are many of them around, certainly, but you don't have to eat them all. Some examples: jam, coffee, wine, sugar, most fizzy drinks, some biscuits and crackers and even a few surprises like small portions of some fruits. These foods generally get in the way of you creating a really excellent diet and we suggest you find alternatives to as many of them as you can. There are many foods which have zero RiskPoints yet offer useful numbers of Life-Points, too. We have listed some of them for your convenience (see free foods, page 114), you can eat these foods whenever you like without clocking up lots of RiskPoints.

Destroy! *The habits that add nothing to your LifePoints rating.*

Target Five

Your diet is weak if you are not eating enough. Does that surprise you? Many people think 'diet' means 'dieting', with all the frenzy of calorie counting that implies. Well, LifePoints – as we hope you realize by now – is different. Calories don't tell you anything about the goodness of food, so we don't use them. And calorie counting keeps 'dieters' in a state of anxiety that deprives them of any pleasure or instinctive awareness of their food. Instead, the LifePoints system uses positive information to help you achieve success and a positive attitude while creating a diet that suits you. As you will see from the Menu and Meal Collections that follow (pages 61 and 71), you don't go hungry using the LifePoints system. You do start to feel well; you do start to enjoy your food again and you can, if you want, lose weight as well.

> Destroy! *The calorie-counting frame of mind; let your diet become a positive experience rather than a worrying, punishing trial of willpower.*

When you have considered each of these five search and destroy missions, we hope you will realize that your diet is easily and readily within your control. With ease and pleasure, you can eat a healthy diet starting immediately and, as we describe below, you are probably much further along that route than you may realize.

THE 80/20 PHENOMENON

When we started developing the LifePoints system, we noticed that in fact most people ate a diet that was approximately 80 per cent good foods – only the remaining 20 per cent needed 'tweaking' to bring it into line with the LifePoints guidelines. We found that making sometimes quite small changes to improve their diet was easier for most people when they understood that *all* of it didn't have to be altered. This is where the LifePoints system is so friendly and positive: as soon as you start using it, you get results.

Our motto is: success by the inch is a cinch . . . by the yard, it's hard. Improving your diet *one food at a time* is the best way to a healthy long-term food control regime. And only the LifePoints system can help you to pinpoint the weak areas in your diet, then easily and quickly select lots of healthy alternatives! Let's demonstrate how LifePoints can work in this way.

When the LifePoints system first broke into the news, we

appeared live on television (and unrehearsed!) to show Nick Owen (of television's *Good Morning with Anne & Nick*) how he could change just 20 per cent of his day's menu to make it a high-LifePoints diet. Here's a LifePoints analysis of Nick's food intake on the day in question. The basic conclusion: although the RiskPoints total seems at first glance to be very high (202) there were really only one or two small changes to make to turn it into a first-class diet.

Meal	Food	RiskPoints ✗	LifePoints ✔
BREAKFAST and 9 a.m. SNACK	Cornflakes	0	16
	with skimmed milk	1	9
	Buttered toast	20	3
	Banana	1	6
TOTAL FOR BREAKFAST and SNACK:		22	34
LUNCH	Ham and avocado, chicken and mayonnaise sandwiches on white buttered bread	129	17
DINNER	Cod in a bag with parsley sauce	26	30
	Peas	0	9
	Sweetcorn	2	5
	Broccoli	1	12
	Mashed potato	22	8
	Wine	0	0
TOTAL DINNER:		51	64
TOTAL FOR DAY:		202	115

This is how we explained the simple changes to Nick: first of all, the LifePoints system divides food into six main groups; we compared Nick's choices to our recommendations for choosing foods from these groups:

Group	We recommend (daily)	Nick chose
Fruit and Fruit Juices	3 servings	1 serving
Cereals, Grains and Pasta	4 servings	3 servings
Vegetables and Vegetable Products	4 servings	5 servings
Legumes, Nuts and Seeds	3 servings	0 servings
Meat, Fish and Dairy	optional	5 servings
Drinks, Desserts, Snacks and Sauces	optional	3 servings

Immediately, Nick saw that he was short on the fruit group and legume group, and a bit heavy on meat, fish and dairy. That told him where to cut back, but it also told him where to add foods that would subsequently boost his LifePoints rating. Here is what we did to revise his diet:

Breakfast and 9 a.m. snack

Let's swap the butter on that toast for a low-fat spread (people often puzzle whether butter or margarine is best for them, but in fact most of them are pretty high in fat. There are so many good-tasting low-fat spreads around today that changing to one shouldn't be a problem).

Does Nick like *yeast extract*? If so, let's put some on his toast (it's a super source of many B vitamins – choose for preference the low-salt versions available). And finally, a glass of *orange*

juice. Now Nick's breakfast/snack rates like this:
Breakfast/9 a.m. snack
✗ RiskPoints 9
✔ LifePoints 54

Lunch

This looks like the sort of meal grabbed by someone who (like many of us) doesn't have time to sit down to lunch. OK, let's give him a few quick snacks he can eat on the run. First, there's a bit of a problem with the sandwich fillings. Two sandwiches are a bit boring for lunch, and variety is one of the most important qualities of a good diet, so we're going to replace one sandwich completely, and slightly change the other one.

Sandwich: avocado and watercress, with low-fat spread and/or low-fat dressing
Baked Potato filled with baked beans (you can get baked potatoes anywhere, Spud-U-Like etc.)
Mixed salad with French dressing
Apricots: dried (a real power food, carry them anywhere!)

Here's what Nick's lunch rated when we'd finished with it:
Lunch
✗ RiskPoints 53
✔ LifePoints 50

Dinner

Not bad! We just changed the mashed potato (often high in fat) to spiced rice to get a new Dinner rating:
Dinner
✗ RiskPoints 30
✔ LifePoints 62

With these rather minor changes we came up with a new LifePoints rating for Nick's day menu:
FULL DAY
✗ RiskPoints 92
✔ LifePoints 166

Not bad! With just a few changes we slashed Nick's RiskPoints in half, boosting his LifePoints without any special effort. Yet, the basic feel and shape of his meals remained the same – something we are sure that Nick approved of. In fact, most of us settle into a way of eating where the look and style of food is dear to us. LifePoints enables you to keep that very personal appeal in your meals whilst lifting them out of nutritional doldrums.

People from all walks of life and with greatly varied lifestyles and eating patterns have found the simple 80/20 changes we suggest just as quick and easy to make as did Nick. Here are some more real-life examples from readers who enjoyed immediate and very positive control of their diets using the LifePoints system:

CASE ONE – SAMANTHA

Samantha's what we call a 'grazer': apart from the evening meal, most of her eating consists of grabbing a quick snack when she can. With two bouncy youngsters to look after, as well as a part-time job to hold down, there's no time for lengthy cooking sessions. LifePoints can really help people like Samantha, because the system allows her to prioritize her food intake according to her personal needs – in her case, maximum nutrition in minimum time. Now, snack foods can often be very fattening, but they don't have to be. With a little tweaking, we can improve her present eating habits enormously – without giving her the 'I'm-on-a-diet' blues! Samantha likes strong, salty and fatty tastes, so we tried to give her strong flavours and satisfying meals.

Samantha's old diet	RiskPoints	LifePoints	Samantha's new LifePoints diet	RiskPoints ✗	LifePoints ✔
BREAKFAST					
2 slices toast with butter	40	3	2 slices toast with yeast extract and low-fat margarine	12	14
Marmalade	0	0	Tea with skimmed milk	1	3
Tea with skimmed milk	1	3	Glass pineapple juice	0	8
LUNCH					
Ham salad sandwich	20	8	Spicy bean pâté salad sandwich	10	23
Packet crisps	24	3	1 oz dried gingko nuts (a bit exotic, but very tasty and why not!)	1	6
Apple	1	1	Banana	1	6
_or_ banana	1	6	Glass carrot juice (so refreshing – buy it in any health food shop)	0	13
AFTERNOON SNACK					
Tea	1	3	Tea	1	3
2 choc biscuits	22	1	Fruit and cereal snack bar	13	40
DINNER					
Spaghetti bolognese	57	31	Lasagne bolognese (made with TVP mince)	10	61
Mixed veg	0	11	Mixed veg	0	11
			½ cup white sauce with herbs	23	7
			Fresh orange	0	6
EVENING SNACK					
2 portions of tortilla chips	36	2	Baked potato with broad bean and broccoli filling (no butter)	13	40
2 tbs sour cream	22	0			
TOTALS	224	66		85	241

As you can see, we've boosted Samantha's nutrient intake by nearly trebling her LifePoints rating, greatly increased her variety (she was weak in all four core food groups) and – best of all – she won't go hungry.

CASE TWO – MELISSA

Melissa is a dieter but calorie counting has failed for her – she's still half a stone heavier than she wants to be – so now's her chance to slim down *and* improve her nutritional intake, both at the same time! There's a bit of Jekyll and Hyde in every dieter, and Melissa's no exception. During the day she single-handedly keeps the crispbread industry going! But after nightfall it's a bit of an orgy! We're going to even things out a bit, to keep her energy levels more constant and to stop those hunger pangs before they start. Melissa's told us that her morning toast and honey is sacrosanct – which is fine, we'll make some changes in other areas. Also, we can greatly improve the variety in her diet (does the word 'boring' presently come to mind?) so as to heighten the pleasure she gets from her food. Diets do not have to be painful!

Melissa's old diet	RiskPoints	LifePoints	Melissa's new LifePoints diet	RiskPoints ✗	LifePoints ✔
BREAKFAST					
2 slices toast with margarine	26	3	2 slices toast with margarine	26	3
Honey	0	0	Honey	0	0
Black tea	0	0	Black tea	0	0
			½ cantaloupe melon	1	10
LUNCH					
Crispbread	0	1	Baked potato with baked beans	1	20
Cucumber	0	1	Cup of diluted yeast extract	0	11
Cup of broth	3	1			
AFTERNOON SNACK					
Apple	1	1	Melon and apricot smoothie	2	27
Black coffee	0	0	Crispbread	0	1
Crispbread	0	1	Bean pâté	0	11
DINNER					
Roast beef	64	18	Cream of mushroom soup	13	16
Roast potatoes	5	9	Baked lemon tempeh (buy tempeh in any health food shop)	23	39
Cabbage	1	5	Heart of gold roasted pumpkin	0	10
Carrots	0	7	Wild rice risotto	3	22
Wine	0	0	Steamed green beans	0	10
			Apple and raspberry pie	6	33
TOTALS	100	47		75	213

Again, we've successfully reduced Melissa's RiskPoints while increasing the variety and quality of the food she eats – quadrupling her LifePoints intake and even adding another course to the evening meal, which now includes a dessert as a bonus!

CASE THREE – JENNY

This is a very sugary, very fatty diet, lacking in food that is alive and fresh. It is also the highest RiskPoints rating we'd seen for a long time (until we saw her husband's, that is!). Our task has been to quarter the RiskPoints while boosting Jenny's LifePoints and including more variety – a number of servings from each of the four essential food groups and fewer from the optional groups. We have kept to Jenny's style of eating – mostly ready-made, snack or convenience foods – but think that maybe she or her husband could learn to cook up a favourite food at home, even if just once a week, to boost their LifePoints.

Jenny's old diet	RiskPoints	LifePoints	Jenny's new LifePoints diet	RiskPoints ✗	LifePoints ✓
BREAKFAST					
3 Shredded Wheat	2	6	1 bowlful 40 % bran flakes	1	32
1 cup semi-skimmed milk	22	14	¾ cup skimmed milk	1	9
Sugar	0	0	1 banana, sliced	1	6
Tea with semi-skimmed milk	12	3	Tea with skimmed milk	1	3
			1 glass orange juice	1	9
MORNING SNACK					
Jam doughnut	39	6	Dried apricots	0	8
1 apple	1	1	Dried figs	2	7
Coffee with semi-skimmed milk	11	7	Carrot juice	0	13
Chocolate bar	35	4	Banana bread made with margarine	15	3
LUNCH					
Corned beef sandwich	21	15	Baked potato with coleslaw	4	14
Crisps	24	3	Mixed salad with low-fat thousand island dressing	4	9
Natural yogurt	0	9	Natural yogurt	0	9
Diet Coke	0	0	Tomato juice	0	6
AFTERNOON SNACK					
Snack bar	35	4	2 bagels (plain, onion, poppy or sesame seed)	4	10
Tea with semi-skimmed milk	12	3	With yeast extract and Bean pâté	0	11
DINNER					
Lasagne	75	34	Ravioli with spinach and cheese filling	41	21
Sweet corn	2	5	Steamed courgettes	0	2
Garlic bread	40	6	Steamed carrots	0	7
			Green beans	0	10
			EVENING SNACK		
			Popcorn, air popped	0	1
TOTALS	331	120		75	201

Let's look immediately at Jenny's husband's diet:

CASE FOUR – NIGEL

Nigel's old diet	RiskPoints	LifePoints	Nigel's new LifePoints diet	RiskPoints ✗	LifePoints ✔
BREAKFAST					
4 Shredded Wheat	2	6	1 bowlful 40 % bran flakes	1	32
1½ cups full-fat milk	74	9	¾ cup skimmed milk	1	9
Sugar	0	0	1 banana, sliced	1	6
Tea with milk and sugar	12	3	Tea with skimmed milk	1	3
			1 glass orange juice	1	9
			2 bagels (plain, onion, poppy or sesame seed)	4	10
			with Bean pâté	0	11
			and yeast extract	0	11
MORNING SNACK					
Tuna salad sandwich	69	29	Vegetable burger in bun with condiments	17	17
6 chocolate wafer bars	342	4	Banana bread with margarine	15	3
1 apple	1	1	Dried figs	2	7
Tea with milk and sugar	12	3	Tomato juice	0	6
LUNCH					
Ham and cheese sandwich	48	20	Baked potato with baked beans, no butter	1	20
Cheese and pickle sandwich	53	15	Dried apricots	0	8
Ham sandwich	17	12	1 apple	1	1
1 nectarine	1	7	Carrot juice	0	13
Tea with milk and sugar	24	3	Tea with skimmed milk	1	3

Case Four – Nigel *contd*

Nigel's old diet	RiskPoints	LifePoints	Nigel's new LifePoints diet	RiskPoints ✗	LifePoints ✔
DINNER					
Lasagne	75	34	Ravioli with spinach and cheese filling	41	21
Sweet corn	2	5	Steamed courgettes	0	2
Garlic bread	40	6	Steamed carrots	0	7
Sponge and custard	24	9	Green beans	0	10
			Sponge with apple sauce	2	4
EVENING SNACK					
Milk chocolate bar	60	4	Muesli bar	12	2
Shortbread biscuits	4	0	Popcorn, air-popped	0	1
TOTALS	860	170		101	216

Nigel and Jenny both needed to reduce their RiskPoints, Nigel especially so. Because Nigel does not wish to reduce his weight, we have allowed him the standard 100 RiskPoints per day, but greatly increased his LifePoints. He works hard physically so we have made especially sure that he will not feel hungry on our suggested diet and we have, as with Jenny, kept his diet sweet by adding fresh and dried fruits in place of sugar. Both Nigel and Jenny needed to spread their food intake over the four essential food groups and we have helped them do this. Both can still pop out to a high-street shop for their lunches. We have kept them eating together in the evening and, in fact, Jenny can join in the evening snack of popcorn if she wishes. As they are a couple, we also tried to include many of the same foods in the rest of their diet, so that they can economize on shopping and any cooking they might do: dried fruits and banana bread, for instance.

WORKING THE 80/20 RULE FOR YOUR OWN DIET
The 80/20 Rule can be enacted in four steps: analyse, highlight, select, adjust. Let's work through them.

When you first start using the LifePoints system you may

wonder how to find the 20 per cent of your diet that is veering off in the wrong direction, and how you can change it easily and quickly. For, no matter how eager you are to improve your health, it is always strenuous to contemplate throwing out a whole lifetime's pattern of buying and preparing food. Well, recognizing that 20 per cent of your diet that's dragging you down is actually very easy. Our first target is variety. When you eat a diet that is full of variety you almost guarantee a diet high in LifePoints. And if you select your variety of foods from the four essential food groups, then you also quite naturally and pain-lessly limit the number of RiskPoints in your diet. Here are the essential food groups and the number of servings we suggest you take from each, every day. Can you recall your intake from each food group based on what you ate yesterday or today? Jot down the totals in the column provided using the listings section of this book if you need to clarify to which group a particular food belongs.

Group	We recommend (daily)	Your diet today
Fruit and Fruit Juices	3 servings	
Cereals, Grains and Pasta	4 servings	
Vegetables and Vegetable Products	4 servings	
Legumes, Nuts and Seeds	3 servings	
Meat, Fish and Dairy	optional	
Drinks, Desserts, Snacks and Sauces	optional	

So the first step is understanding the importance of variety and knowing how much variety you actually get or don't get in your present way of eating. Once you see a gap – as did Nick when he noticed he ate no legumes – you can easily and quickly fill it by referring to the foods listed in the Legumes, Nuts and Seeds section. It's as simple as that!

The blank form that follows is your Daily Food Planner. We would like you to write on it every food item you eat today or tomorrow. Then, at the end of the day, browse through the food listings and note the RiskPoints and LifePoints associated with each of those foods. At the same time, learn to which of the six food groups each food belongs and tick the appropriate column.

Now simply add up the RiskPoints, the LifePoints and the ticks in each of the six food groups. Instantly, you have a clear profile of your diet. Now you can see for yourself where your diet is good and where it lets you down. And because you can see so clearly, you are able to make small changes *right now* that will bring that wayward 20 per cent of your diet back into line.

One more thing before we move on: after a very short time analysing your diet in this way, you will find that the LifePoints system has helped you to reawaken your instincts for good food! Your taste for very fatty food will diminish; you will quite naturally and almost without thought wish for the tastes and food items that will do you good. We have called the first week the Lift-Off; by the third or fourth week you will be enjoying the ease and naturalness of food selection we describe.

THE LIFEPOINTS DAILY FOOD PLANNER

FOOD	RiskPoints ✗	LifePoints ✔	TICK FOOD GROUP					
			Fruit and Fruit Juices	Cereals, Grains and Pasta	Vegetables and Vegetable Products	Legumes, Nuts and Seeds	Meat, Fish and Dairy	Drinks, Desserts Snacks and Sauces

Now you have all the tools you need to improve your diet. Here they are again, in shorthand, to help you with your Lift-Off:

● Use the Food Planner to analyse your diet for two or three days – even a week – until you get a feel for where your particular diet weaknesses lie. This period of time will also enable you to read through the food listings at least once and to get acquainted with the LifePoints and RiskPoints associated with your favourite foods.

   The next step is, of course, to select foods that will replace those which bring too many RiskPoints into your diet as well as those which fill you up without adding much of anything at all to your diet. Here's how:

● Find the foods in your completed Food Planner that are highest in RiskPoints and highlight them or make a list of them.
● Now find the essential food group or groups from which you are not currently eating sufficient servings.
● Select new foods which will add servings to the food group or groups needing them, as well as fit the rôle of a high-RiskPoints food you have highlighted. For instance, highlighting spaghetti in four cheese sauces (a whacking great 384 RiskPoints) you are suddenly left without a main course for that dinner. You need another serving from the legumes food group so you can keep the spaghetti but serve it with a TVP bolognaise sauce (made with soya bean mince instead of meat). Instantly, you have met all your requirements happily and without loss of time, flavour or pleasure.
● Finally, you may adjust your food selection to suit more completely your tastes, your budget, your schedule. This adjustment is necessarily gradual but you may be surprised at how natural it feels to you – as though you'd been craving your new food choices for a very long time.

YOUR TRANSITION TO THE LIFEPOINTS LIFESTYLE

To make your transition even more comfortable, we have designed some meals and menus that will do the thinking for you. First, we offer the Menu Collection, seven day-menus that are high in LifePoints and rate no more than 100 RiskPoints. Each of these menus is fairly conventional in style as well as being easy to purchase or prepare. We have designed them to be as close to an unchanged diet as possible so that you can perhaps see your own style of eating represented somewhere among them. Choose one of these menus for each day of the seven-day LifePoints Lift-Off. You may try each one of the seven or rotate, using those three, four or five that most appeal to you.

If none of them appeals, or if you wish to have greater choice during each day, please turn to our Meal Collection on page 71. Here we offer our second collection – this time a list of seven each of breakfasts, lunches, dinners, morning snacks and after-noon snacks. You simply select one from each of these groups to compose your day's menu. This collection lets you experiment a little more than the Menu Collection but still keeps your LifePoints wonderfully high and your RiskPoints no more than 100.

You may use the Meal Collection or the Menu Collection for all or part of the LifePoints Lift-Off period, but please don't mix the two. Also, please try and adhere to the suggested foods as closely as possible, especially avoiding foods that will send the Risk-Points rating soaring. Obvious 'culprits' include butter, cheese and fried foods; less obvious foods will become apparent to you as you familiarize yourself with the food listings. Also, study the tips on page 101 to help you avoid 'fat traps' and other food mistakes. If you wish to extend the Lift-Off period to more than one week, these two collections will provide you with ample guidance to do so.

ANY QUESTIONS?

How long should I try it for?
A two-week trial should be enough time for you to feel comfortable with LifePoints and to start to feel an appreciable benefit.

How much weight can I lose?
If you're using the LifePoints system to lose weight, you should be prepared for something that works rather more gradually than the 'thin thighs in thirty days' school of thought that we've come

to expect from diet books. In 1991 the results of the world's longest controlled human-feeding study ever to be undertaken were published.[10] Scientifically speaking, it was a beautifully designed study.[11] Thirteen women aged between 22 and 56 were randomly put into one of two groups. The first ate a low-fat diet (at about the 125 RiskPoints limit) while the second group ate a control diet (moderately calorie-restricted but not low in fat). Both groups ate the same type of food, but the low-fat group ate reduced-fat versions (e.g. low-fat yogurt instead of regular). Significantly, although the low-fat group could eat as much food as they wanted to, they actually chose to consume about 250 fewer calories a day. After eleven weeks, the subjects were given a complete break for seven weeks (a so-called 'washout' period) and then the tables were turned – the low-fat group went on to the control diet and the former control group ate low-fat. This sort of study is called a 'crossover' study, and is a powerful way of eliminating bias and individual idiosyncrasies.

The results were very encouraging. The women on the low-fat diet had lost twice as much weight as those on the calorie-controlled diet – about ½ lb per week, 2½kg in 11 weeks. Now, of course, people differ very greatly in their degree of weight loss – after all, we're all different! As the scientists wrote:

> There is a great deal of evidence that conscious reduction in the amount of food consumed results in rapid losses of body weight; but almost invariably this lost weight is regained. Reductions in the fat content of the diet with no limitation on the amount of food consumed may lead to a more permanent weight loss than can be achieved through [conventional] dieting.

Finally, we want to add one last point about the way weight loss may occur on LifePoints. We strongly suspect that much of today's overeating is caused not by gluttony, but simply by the body's natural quest for a highly nutritious diet. Wouldn't it be ironic if, in the quest for optimum nutrition, our bodies' instincts are actually precipitating one of today's major threats to our health? Of course, the LifePoints system can help here, too, by guiding us to the most nutritious foods.

What about alcohol?

If you're dieting to lose weight, then alcohol isn't on the menu. Not only does it supply you with calories without any nutritional value (so-called 'empty' calories), but it can also alter your body chemistry so as to temporarily reduce your natural ability to burn off fat.[12] At other times, we suggest you restrict your consumption to no more than two glasses of red wine per day. In most countries, high dietary intakes of saturated fats are strongly associated with high coronary heart disease death rates. Some regions of France, however, appear to be an exception to this rule: they have low heart disease death rates despite high-fat diets. This paradox may be due to the antioxidant phenolic compounds which red wine contains (and, as we all know, the French *do* drink red wine). No other alcohol has this effect.

What about 'double-zero' foods?

Browsing through the foods in the Counter, you'll notice that some of them have no LifePoints and no RiskPoints; these are double-zero foods. Don't make the mistake of thinking that they can be eaten abundantly. People who are used to counting calories occasionally confuse the LifePoints system with their previous dietary regime. It's not the same at all! Double-zero foods are empty foods and have little place in your diet strategy. Remember, you have two objectives:

1   To achieve a high LifePoints score.
2   To keep your RiskPoints within your chosen limit.

Double-zero foods do *not* help you to achieve your prime dietary goal of a healthy LifePoints score. In fact, they are counter-productive, because they make it less likely that you'll have the appetite to eat higher-scoring foods during the day. The Life-Points system helps you *prioritize* your food intake. Double-zero foods are very low priority.

Is there any need to take food supplements?

Certain groups in the population have enhanced nutritional needs. In today's society, where food is so plentiful, it may seem strange to think that under-nutrition can occur at all, but the evidence shows that it can. Although you can substantially increase your overall nutrient intake by following the LifePoints system, you should still be aware that some nutrients are not particularly easy to obtain from day-to-day food sources. In particular, there can be a real need, especially at certain times of life, to take in supplementary amounts of the following nutrients:

- *Calcium:* if your dietary intake of this vital mineral is consistently too low bone degeneration may occur. Many people incorrectly suppose that the consumption of copious amounts of dairy produce is the only way to prevent bone-depleting afflictions such as osteoporosis. This isn't true – strangely enough, people who eat meat and dairy products are more at risk of bone loss than non-meat eaters. Good plant food sources of calcium include blackstrap molasses, sesame seeds, tofu, green leafy vegetables such as collards or cabbage, almonds and carob flour. Calcium is best absorbed when you have adequate vitamin D in your body (sunlight is a good source) and when there's plenty of boron in the diet (available in apples and other fresh fruits and vegetables).
- *Iron:* generally conserved well by the body (90 per cent of the 3 to 5 grams in our bodies is continually recycled); the major cause of iron depletion is loss of blood itself – as in menstruation. Women of childbearing age should therefore take care to eat good dietary sources, which include blackstrap molasses, pumpkin and squash seeds, spirulina, many fortified breakfast cereals, quinoa, dried mixed fruit, wheat germ and kidney beans. Foods which contain vitamin C (e.g. fresh fruit and vegetables) will considerably increase your absorption. Several factors can significantly reduce absorption of iron, among them tea (the tannin forms insoluble iron compounds) and the food preservative EDTA. Both of these can reduce assimilation by as much as 50 per cent.
- *Vitamin B12:* if you are eating a diet composed exclusively of plant-based foods (i.e. from the first four groups only) make sure you sometimes consume a good source of vitamin B12, such as fortified breakfast cereal, fortified soya milk, yeast extract or fermented food such as tempeh.

Do I have to make allowances for the freshness of food?

Yes, you do. The level of nutrition you receive from your diet depends not only on what food you choose to eat, but also on how you store and cook it. This provides at least three opportunities for nutrient loss. If you lead a hectic, demanding life you need these nutrients even more and therefore need to know how you can safeguard them. So please, read and take to heart the advice which follows:

- The more a foodstuff is processed, the greater the loss of natural nutrients. So buy only unprocessed wholefoods.
- If possible buy organic food, preferably from local producers. Organic foods are more likely to have their nutrients intact and if they are from local producers they will not have been in long storage during transit. Nutrients decay with time – so eat close to the soil! Also, the risk of pesticide residue is remote. Pesticides are poisons – their basic purpose is to kill. In an ideal world, pesticides are not supposed to leave any residue on food by the time it's ready for us to eat. But considerable evidence indicates that the food we eat *can* be tainted with pesticide residue, even if it's been washed many times. Herbicides are often absorbed directly into the system of the plant itself, so that it is impossible to get rid of them simply by washing.

Thankfully, many supermarket chains have now started to stock organic produce. So what is organic food? The Soil Association states:

Organic food is produced responsibly, taking account of the needs of consumers, farm animals and the environment. Organic farmers produce food which:

- Is grown without artificial pesticides and fertilisers
- Tastes good rather than just looks good
- Is never irradiated
- Contains no artificial hormones, genetically manipulated organisms or unnecessary medication
- Is not over-processed to remove the goodness
- Does not contain flavourings, dyes and other additives

- Is nutritious, living food which promotes positive health and wellbeing.

Organic food is also better for the environment. Intensive agriculture is responsible for about 50 per cent of all water pollution (such as high nitrate levels). It has been clearly established that modern biological-organic farming methods lead both to lower leaching of nitrates into the water supply and to lower nitrate content in vegetables.

If you can't afford to eat organic food all the time (and it can be very expensive), at least try to make sure that your children eat as organically as possible. Children are much more vulnerable than adults to the toxic effects of chemical residue.

Now, here are a few more tips to maximize the nutritional bang in your food:

- Check the use-by date. Old produce will have suffered severe nutritional decay. Shopkeepers always put older stock at the front of the display – so rearrange their display and buy from the back.
- Canning and bottling reduces the levels of vitamin C, thiamin and folic acid. Vitamin C loss continues during storage. if you have to buy canned food, do not keep it overlong. Although it may be safe to eat, its nutrients may be severely depleted.
- Avoid foods which contain sulphur dioxide as a preservative – they will have almost entirely lost their thiamin (vitamin B1) content.
- Freeze-dried foods are relatively good since there is no heating to deplete nutrients.
- Frozen foods suffer some thiamin and vitamin C loss. However, the loss is less than in fresh food which has been kept for a number of days. If shopping for fresh food is a problem for you, frozen foods are probably the next best alternative, but be extra careful not to overcook them.
- Choose unrefined monounsaturated oils – preferably olive oil – for cooking. Pure, refined polyunsaturated oils turn rancid more easily.
- Don't buy tinned goods which are damaged – no matter how good a bargain they appear to be. Small cracks in the lining inside the cans affect the contents, which will certainly affect

the delicate vitamins and other nutrients and may even cause the food itself to turn bad.

- Store oils, fats and oily foods like cheeses and shelled nuts in the refrigerator. This will help to slow down the process of oxidation which turns them rancid.

- Vitamin C, thiamin, riboflavin and folic acid all decay quickly in air. Once vegetables are harvested, the damaged tissues release an enzyme which starts to destroy the vitamin C. Blanching inhibits the enzyme, which is why freezing fresh vegetables is much better than keeping them unfrozen and eating them many days later.

- Vegetables lose around 70 per cent of their folic acid content within three days if they are stored in daylight. Store vegetables in the refrigerator until you are ready to use them, or freeze them straight away.

- Store grains and cereals whole and in a dry, cool place.

- Cooking is generally harmful to the nutrients in food. However, it also changes starches, proteins and some vitamins into accessible forms for us, as well as releasing nutrients in some foods which are otherwise bound in, like the amino acid tryptophan in cornmeal. Cooking is necessary for other foods, to destroy toxic substances such as those found in soybeans and kidney beans. Cooking also makes some foods – like meat – palatable to eat. However, there are ways in which you can reduce the nutrient loss in foods during the cooking process.

- Pressure cooking is perhaps the best way to reduce nutrient loss. Invest in a non-aluminium pressure cooker which, because of the reduced cooking times, will also reduce energy consumption and therefore the size of your fuel bills.

- After pressure cooking, steaming and microwave cooking are the next-healthiest options. Buying a steamer is obviously a lot cheaper than buying a microwave oven! Further down the list are:

    Boiling
    Grilling
    Stir frying (at high temperature where the fat seals in the nutrients)
    Sautéing
    Deep frying.

- If you cook with fat don't let it become so hot that it starts to smoke. At this temperature the essential fatty acid linoleic acid is destroyed immediately.
- Fats which have been used for cooking once must be discarded since the linoleic acid and vitamins A and C will have been lost.
- If you boil food, do so for the minimum amount of time and then use the water for stock afterwards. The fragile water-soluble vitamins, as well as some minerals, leach into cooking water, which is why soups are so nutritious.
- Don't add bicarbonate of soda to cooking water, even if you see it recommended in cooking pulses. It destroys valuable B vitamins.
- Prepare food immediately before cooking – remember that vitamin C is destroyed once cells are damaged in vegetables – and, for the same reason, try not to chop them too finely. Scrubbing vegetables is better than peeling them.
- Once they have been prepared, steam or cook the vegetables in ready boiling water straight away.
- Use pans with close-fitting lids and avoid using copper pans, which encourage oxidation and vitamin C loss.
- Once food is cooked, eat it straight away. Keeping it warm will only result in further nutrient loss, which is why eating out too frequently may be less than healthy for you.

If you lead a hectic lifestyle and consider that you don't have time for some of the advice given above, think again. The life you lead is totally dependent on a good nutritional support system, without which you're just running on empty. And you can only do that for so long. Shopping regularly for fresh foods can appear to present a problem – if you don't attach a very high priority to it. But just think – no sensible person buys a Rolls-Royce then tries to run it on two-star petrol! It's the same with your body – the better the fuel, the better the performance you'll receive.

Do I have to follow the measurements given?

The more accurate you can be with your measurements, the better the system will work for you. To make things as easy as possible, most of the foods are listed in common measurements (a cup, a slice, and so on). Remember, we want you to eat as widely as possible. Do you know what the prime cause of malnutrition is? Most people in the West often erroneously believe that it's lack of food, but that's not true. The principal cause of malnutrition is lack of *variety* in food. A monotonous diet is a dangerous diet. So choose your food as widely as possible!

Can't I just subtract the RiskPoints from the LifePoints to produce one simple number?

In a word, no. They measure two completely different aspects of a food's worth, and it is not possible to combine them meaningfully. However, we think having two numbers is actually superior to having one. This is why: one number tells you very little about the good and bad ingredients in a foodstuff. It doesn't allow you to make a mental picture of that food, nor does it allow you to see how and where that food might fit into your diet. Having two numbers allows you to get more of a *feel* for the food concerned – which is what we want. When you've used the system for a day or two, you'll see what we mean.

What happens if I exceed my daily RiskPoints?

Your first priority is to choose good food to eat. And that should be fun! Don't feel dejected if you exceed your RiskPoints limit from time to time – it happens! Just try gradually to get those RiskPoints down. It may take some time to re-educate your tastebuds, particularly if you're used to a high-fat diet. The LifePoints system is a tool; use it as you would any other to achieve your success over a period of time. And remember, 'success by the inch is a cinch – by the yard, it's hard!'

How can I put together meals and recipes using Life-Points?

Easily! Remember, go for variety. Choose from all of the first four groups. When you've chosen a food from one group, go to another for your next food choice. As far as recipes are concerned, we'd like you to try *LifePoints Cookbook*, which shows you just how easy it is to produce delicious foods and meals using the system. And it gives you over 150 quick, easy and economical recipes too!

I really go to pieces at Christmas and other special occasions.

We know – these occasions are full of family and social pressures and the appeal of traditional foods. That's why we wrote *LifePoints Cookbook*, which has plenty of ideas for you to consider for celebrations and entertaining.

What should I do when I feel weak-willed and want to eat something with a no-no RiskPoint number?

Choose something else! There are plenty of foods with respectable LifePoints numbers and zero or few RiskPoints. Remember – you're in control! You eat what you want to eat. The LifePoints system is all about taking charge of your own diet. If you want to choose bad food, then that's your decision – we're not going to nag you! But here's a tip: immediately you sense that feeling, take out a notepad and write down exactly what you want to do, and put its RiskPoints number beside it in BIG DIGITS. Now look at what you have written. Your inclination to do that thing is guaranteed to diminish.

I always start diets but then get fed up cooking two meals – one for myself and another for my family.

This is a really common problem. Since preparing two sets of meals is almost impossible to do for any length of time, you must sit down with your family and tell them about the LifePoints system. Then tell them that it is difficult to make two meals and that this has, in the past, caused you many problems with diets. If they're worth their salt, they will come up with a number of ideas that may help share and solve this problem. They may decide that they want to eat healthily too – or someone might even volunteer to help you with the food!

I'm a fast eater. When I finish my first serving, my family aren't even halfway through theirs, so I usually take another serving just to keep them company. I know this has caused a lot of my weight problems, but how can I slow down?

There are a number of simple, unobtrusive little techniques you can use to help you eat more slowly.

- Don't cut your food into pieces all at once (if it needs cutting). Instead, cut one bite-sized piece at a time, eat it, then cut the next piece.
- Take a spoon or fork full of food, then put your fork down on the side of your plate while you chew that mouthful. Don't pick up the next spoonful until you have swallowed the first.
- Buy a set of pretty cloth napkins and use one at each meal. Wipe your mouth frequently during the meal to help slow you down.
- Take a slow, deep breath in and out between each mouthful of food. This will take the hurry out of eating as well as keep you relaxed.
- With all of this slow eating, you might think your food will go cold. Warm your plate before serving to prevent this. Also, take small portions of food so that the rest remains in the hot serving dish.

I use a lot of oil and fat in cooking and I've got used to the flavour. What is a good substitute for all this fat?

Cut the fat in cooking to an absolute minimum. Ignore the fat included in the recipes you use and, when it seems essential, try cutting the amount listed in half.

- Blend a little tomato or tandoori paste with 2 fl. oz (60ml) water and pour into your pan. Place over a high flame and when the liquid bubbles, add your vegetables and stir frequently. This is what we call the 'LifePoints Sauté' method – the liquid replaces the fat normally used in a sauté. You will be surprised at how tasty this is.
- Put the fat in serving dishes on the table instead of in your cooking. Each person can then add fat to their own meal. If you are faced with blocks of fat and jugs of oil, you will use very little on your food – it just isn't appetizing.
- Try *LifePoints Cookbook*!

I have a really sweet tooth that always gets the better of me. What can I do to stop myself eating sweet things?

There's nothing at all wrong with eating sweet foods such as fresh fruit. Use LifePoints to find the best! But as far as puddings and desserts are concerned, a sweet tooth is really a bully that always wants to have its own way. You will have to turn it gradually into a more respectable creature. Start by depriving your sweet tooth, a little at a time, of what it wants. Instead of a chocolate bar, eat some dried figs or raisins. Instead of sugary tea or coffee, drink it unsugared with a piece of sugarless oat cake to give you slow-release energy. Next, try retraining your sweet tooth to become a sour tooth. The flavours are equally strong, but the effects are wonderfully different. Every time you want a sweet 'injection', chew on a wedge of lemon, take a sip of cider vinegar in water, or eat a gherkin. Finally, give yourself time to break yourself of the sweet habit. If you have one or two bad days, don't give up. Keep going and you will succeed.

PART THREE: THE LIFEPOINTS MENU COLLECTION

All the meals which follow may be prepared at home. We suggest you read through The LifePoints Shopper's Guide for some tips on how to do your shopping so that all the high-LifePoints, low-RiskPoints foods are there in your cupboard when you need them. We'll also give tips on what dishes to prepare at the weekend – the Bean Pâté, for instance – so that you can use them all week without added fuss.

Although we have altered breakfast, lunch and dinner for each menu, we have provided a morning and afternoon snack that is the same for each of the seven menus listed. See page 114 for a list of 'free' foods – high in LifePoints but rating zero RiskPoints – these foods can be eaten freely in addition to those listed in the menus. Please note, however, that free foods are not the same as double-zero foods – those which provide no LifePoints either. Certainly there are times when double-zero foods are taken (the wine and coffee offered in a meal out, for instance), but we do not encourage this as it adds nothing to the value of your diet.

MENU ONE
This menu will suit you on those days when you want to feel full all the time. Breakfast is quick and easy to make and very sustaining right through the morning. Lunch is readily available in this form from many cafés, sandwich bars and quick-order restaurants. Only dinner requires a bit of your time, and not very much of that: lasagne that needs no precooking is a timesaver for this dish, and when the lasagne is cooked, pop the apples in the oven. They'll be ready by the time you've finished your main course.

Breakfast
porridge made with skimmed milk and added raisins
a glass of orange juice
a banana
tea or coffee with milk

Morning snack
1 carrot, cut into sticks
1 stalk celery, cut into sticks
approximately 3 oz Bean Pâté
a glass of tomato juice

Lunch
baked potato with margarine and baked beans
a mixed side salad (no fish, meat or cheese) with low-fat French
dressing
a French roll
tinned fruit salad
a glass of carrot juice

Afternoon snack
a handful each of dried apricots and dates
a glass of mineral water

Dinner
a starter of half a cantaloupe melon
followed by steamed asparagus over radicchio with low-fat
thousand island dressing
and lasagne made with soya mince
a glass of pineapple juice
matzos spread with Bean Pâté
after which baked apples with oat and raisin filling (no butter)

Today's total
✗ RiskPoints 76
✔ LifePoints 233

MENU TWO
Start your day with a nearly traditional cooked English breakfast:
only the fried egg and 75 RiskPoints are missing! With a bit of
friendly explanation, you could even get your hotel or local café
to make this version for you. Lunch is another meal which is
available on the run, though you may need to supply your own
dried fruits, while dinner is filling, exotic and easy either to make
at home or to order from a Moroccan or Middle Eastern
restaurant.

Breakfast
½ tin baked beans on toast, no butter
grilled tomato
meatless sausage
wholewheat toast spread with margarine and yeast extract
a glass of orange juice
tea or coffee with milk

Morning snack
1 carrot, cut into sticks
a stalk celery, cut into sticks
approximately 3 oz Bean Pâté
a glass of tomato juice

Lunch
vegetable burger in a bun with condiments and lettuce (no cheese)
with a mixed side salad (no fish, meat or cheese)
with low-fat French dressing or ketchup
a glass of carrot juice
a handful each of dried apricots and figs

Afternoon snack
a handful each of dried apricots and dates
a glass of mineral water

Dinner
a starter of gazpacho served with matzos
followed by couscous with chickpea and vegetable stew
steamed spinach
baked squash
after which half a cantaloupe melon filled with fresh grapes

Today's total
✗ RiskPoints 89
✔ LifePoints 211

MENU THREE
Here we offer a slightly lighter collection of meals, though still very sustaining and satisfying. Breakfast is probably in your

cupboard already and is virtually no effort; lunch is fresh and uplifting – easy to pack yourself or order from a restaurant, pub or sandwich bar. Even dinner could be brought home in little tubs from your favourite deli – just cook up the spaghetti while you slide into your slippers.

Breakfast
Raisin Bran cereal with semi-skimmed milk and sliced banana
a glass of orange juice
a toasted bagel spread with yeast extract
tea or coffee with milk

Morning snack
1 carrot, cut into sticks
1 stalk celery, cut into sticks
approximately 3 oz Bean Pâté
a glass of tomato juice

Lunch
a sandwich of Bean Pâté, watercress and beansprouts
a mixed side salad (no fish, meat or cheese)
with low-fat thousand island dressing
a glass of carrot juice
a fresh apple

Afternoon snack
a handful each of dried apricots and dates
a glass of mineral water

Dinner
a starter of pineapple juice
followed by spaghetti in simple tomato sauce
a side salad of steamed broccoli and broad beans, grated carrot
and diced onion with low-fat French dressing
after which a bowlful of fresh raspberries

Today's total
✘ RiskPoints 79
✔ LifePoints 226

MENU FOUR

We know that many people eat like this all the time, but more likely for you, this is simply a day when you get breakfast in bed. We did this just to show it could be done (we all have our moments); however, the croissant wields 50 RiskPoints all by itself so you only get one and please don't have this breakfast very often. Now pull yourself into shape and enjoy a slightly Greek-style menu for the rest of the day.

Breakfast
one plain croissant
a glass of orange juice
tea or coffee with milk

Morning snack
1 carrot, cut into sticks
1 stalk celery, cut into sticks
approximately 3 oz Bean Pâté
a glass of tomato juice

Lunch
toasted pitta bread filled with mixed salad (no fish, meat or cheese)
with one falafel and low-fat French dressing
a glass of carrot juice
a handful each of dried apricots and dates

Afternoon snack
a handful each of dried apricots and dates
a glass of mineral water

Dinner
a starter of fresh mango
followed by fresh spinach and chickpeas stir fried with yeast extract, freshly ground black pepper, garlic and onion
served over steamed white rice
after which fruit sorbet
and a glass of pineapple juice

Today's total
✘ RiskPoints 81
✔ LifePoints 176

Menu Five

This menu is an ideal one to follow when you are away from home for every meal of the day. The breakfast can be ordered in any hotel; the lunch is a perfect salad bar meal. Dinner is slightly Mexican in its feel – an increasingly popular style of cooking in restaurants, pubs, hotels and at dinner parties. Simply avoid butter on the sweet corn and cheese on the burrito.

Breakfast
Corn Flakes or Rice Krispies with skimmed milk
a glassful of grapefruit juice
toasted bagel spread with yeast extract or Bean Pâté
tea or coffee with milk

Morning snack
1 carrot, cut into sticks
1 stalk celery, cut into sticks
approximately 3 oz Bean Pâté
a glass of tomato juice

Lunch
a large salad platter of coleslaw, cold baked beans, mixed salad (no fish, meat or cheese) with low-fat French dressing, sauer-kraut, sweet pickle and rice salad with fresh garden peas
a glass of orange juice

Afternoon snack
a handful each of dried apricots and dates
a glass of mineral water

Dinner
a starter of boiled corn on the cob with low-fat French dressing instead of butter
followed by burrito with beans, salad and alfalfa sprouts
a glass of vegetable juice cocktail
after which half a cantaloupe melon

Today's total
✘ RiskPoints 81
✔ LifePoints 197

MENU SIX

Some people find it difficult to break their breakfast habits and this menu shows that you can still eat within the 100 RiskPoints limit and have your omelette too. But it costs you! Breakfast alone uses up 60 RiskPoints. We follow on with a light lunch and a fairly traditional Italian-style dinner and hope you will gradually try other breakfasts so you can experience some of the more exciting lunch and dinner options.

Breakfast
2-egg omelette
wholewheat toast with margarine
a glass of orange juice
tea or coffee with milk

Morning snack
1 carrot, cut into sticks
1 stalk celery, cut into sticks
approximately 3 oz Bean Pâté
a glass of tomato juice

Lunch
a cup of black bean soup
rice cakes or crispbreads spread with Bean Pâté
topped with sliced tomato, sliced cucumber and watercress
a glass of carrot juice
a small carton of low-fat fruit yogurt
a banana

Afternoon snack
a handful each of dried apricots and dates
a glass of mineral water

Dinner
a starter of mixed salad (no fish, meat or cheese) with low-fat Italian dressing

a French roll
a glass of pineapple juice
followed by linguine in spiced tomato and mushroom sauce
after which fresh raspberries or blackberries

Today's total
✗ RiskPoints 78
✔ LifePoints 165

Menu Seven
Muesli can be made without nuts, of course, and the RiskPoints rating will be reduced as a result. This is a robust menu which will enable you gently and gradually to get into the LifePoints habit.

Breakfast
muesli made with nuts, added currants and sliced banana, with skimmed milk
a glass of orange juice
tea or coffee with milk

Morning snack
1 carrot, cut into sticks
1 stalk celery, cut into sticks
approximately 3 oz Bean Pâté
a glass of tomato juice

Lunch
a fresh orange
½ tin baked beans on toast spread with yeast extract (no butter)
with vegetable burger patty, grilled tomato and mushrooms
a glass of vegetable juice cocktail

Afternoon snack
a handful each of dried apricots and dates
a glass of mineral water

Dinner
a starter of half a cantaloupe melon
followed by mixed salad (no fish, meat or cheese) with steamed

asparagus, low-fat Italian dressing and breadstick
Risotto alla piemontese
after which a plate of fresh grapes

Today's total
✘ RiskPoints 96
✔ LifePoints 184

PART FOUR: THE LIFEPOINTS MEAL COLLECTION

Here is our second collection: meal and snack menus which you may combine as you wish to create your own day-menu. Simply select one breakfast, one morning snack, one lunch, one afternoon snack and one dinner from the seven listed for each meal and snack time. Try to vary your day-menus as much as possible during the Lift-Off period so that you get a feel for the range of foods and dishes which provide a high LifePoints rating. Over time, you will develop new favourites and your taste in food will change to enable you to experiment comfortably with yet more foods and dishes new to you.

We have designed these meals and snacks so that they have an approximate upper limit of RiskPoints, as follows:

- Breakfast maximum 25 RiskPoints
- Morning snack maximum 10 RiskPoints
- Lunch maximum 25 RiskPoints
- Afternoon snack maximum 10 RiskPoints
- Dinner maximum 30 RiskPoints.

Following these guidelines has ensured that the day-menus you compile will keep within the 100 RiskPoints limit.

BREAKFASTS

Breakfast One
a glass of orange juice
muesli made with nuts, with skimmed milk
a banana
herbal tea or black tea or coffee
✗ RiskPoints 22
✔ LifePoints 29

Breakfast Two
a glass of pineapple juice
porridge made with added raisins and skimmed milk
tea or coffee with milk
✗ RiskPoints 18
✔ LifePoints 29

Breakfast Three
a glass of grapefruit juice
GrapeNuts cereal with skimmed milk
toasted bagel with low-fat margarine and yeast extract or Bean
Pâté
tea or coffee with milk
✗ RiskPoints 19
✔ LifePoints 60

Breakfast Four
a glass of pineapple juice
½ tin baked beans on toast, no butter
grilled tomato, mushrooms and meatless sausage
herbal tea or black tea or coffee
✗ RiskPoints 16
✔ LifePoints 43

Breakfast Five
a glass of orange juice
toasted crumpet with low-fat margarine and yeast extract or Bean
Pâté
plain, low-fat yogurt with sliced banana
herbal tea or black tea or coffee
✗ RiskPoints 16
✔ LifePoints 40

Breakfast Six
a glass of pineapple juice
Raisin Bran cereal with sliced banana and skimmed milk
tea or coffee with milk
✗ RiskPoints 15
✔ LifePoints 58

Breakfast Seven
a glass of orange juice
a fruit salad of 1 banana, raspberries, 1 pear, half a cantaloupe melon
a slice of wholewheat or granary toast with low-fat margarine
tea or coffee with milk
✘ RiskPoints 23
✔ LifePoints 39

MORNING SNACKS

Morning Snack One
a glass of pineapple juice
a handful of dried apricots
a small tub of plain, low-fat yogurt
✘ RiskPoints 8
✔ LifePoints 24

Morning Snack Two
a glass of tomato juice
a sandwich with Bean pâté or yeast extract and alfalfa sprouts
a handful of dates
✘ RiskPoints 10
✔ LifePoints 41

Morning Snack Three
a glass of carrot juice
a cup of sauerkraut on a toasted bagel
a slice of raisin bread
a banana
✘ RiskPoints 5
✔ LifePoints 41

Morning Snack Four
a glass of vegetable juice cocktail
a small slice of pizza with tomato sauce, olives and no cheese
a handful each of dried figs and apricots
✘ RiskPoints 10
✔ LifePoints 32

Morning Snack Five
a glass of orange juice
chunky vegetable soup with matzos
✘ RiskPoints 10
✔ LifePoints 20

Morning Snack Six
a glass of vegetable juice cocktail
coleslaw over a toasted bagel
a small tub of low-fat fruit yogurt
✘ RiskPoints 10
✔ LifePoints 26

Morning Snack Seven
a glass of orange juice
a toasted bagel with yeast extract or Bean Pâté
tinned fruit salad with a small tub of low-fat fruit yogurt
✘ RiskPoints 8
✔ LifePoints 39

LUNCHES

Lunch One
a glass of vegetable juice cocktail
toasted pitta bread filled with mixed salad (no fish, meat or cheese), a falafel, olives and low-fat thousand island dressing
a handful of dried figs
✘ RiskPoints 18
✔ LifePoints 34

Lunch Two
a glass of orange juice
a small slice of pizza with tomato sauce and olives, no cheese with mixed salad (no fish, meat or cheese) and low-fat Italian dressing
half a cantaloupe melon and a small tub of plain low-fat yogurt
✘ RiskPoints 21
✔ LifePoints 46

Lunch Three

a glass of soya milk blended with one banana into a milkshake
a sandwich with Bean Pâté and alfalfa sprouts
a slice of raisin bread
✗ RiskPoints 24
✔ LifePoints 36

Lunch Four

a glass of orange juice
a vegetable burger in a bun with condiments and lettuce
mixed salad (no fish, meat or cheese) with low-fat French dressing or ketchup
a handful each of dried apricots, figs and raisins or currants
✗ RiskPoints 22
✔ LifePoints 56

Lunch Five

a glass of pineapple juice
a bowl of leek and potato soup
toasted bagel with yeast extract or Bean Pâté
half a cantaloupe melon
✗ RiskPoints 23
✔ LifePoints 46

Lunch Six

a glass of orange juice
a baked potato with baked beans, no butter
mixed salad (no fish, meat or cheese) with low-fat French dressing
a slice of banana bread (made with margarine) topped with sliced banana
✗ RiskPoints 20
✔ LifePoints 47

Lunch Seven
a glass of pineapple juice
toasted pitta bread with hummus
mixed salad (no fish, meat or cheese) dressed with lemon juice
a handful of dried apricots
✘ RiskPoints 26
✔ LifePoints 45

Afternoon Snacks

Afternoon Snack One
a glass of orange juice
a cup of apple sauce
toasted bagel with low-fat margarine
✘ RiskPoints 7
✔ LifePoints 20

Afternoon Snack Two
a glass of carrot juice
matzos spread with Bean Pâté
fresh grapes
✘ RiskPoints 0
✔ LifePoints 28

Afternoon Snack Three
a glass of tomato juice
baked potato with coleslaw
✘ RiskPoints 3
✔ LifePoints 20

Afternoon Snack Four
a glass of orange juice
toasted bagel with low-fat margarine
a bowlful of fresh raspberries or blackberries
✘ RiskPoints 8
✔ LifePoints 25

Afternoon Snack Five
a glass of vegetable juice cocktail
a toasted bagel spread with Bean pâté

topped with sliced tomato and cucumber
a slice of raisin bread
✘ RiskPoints 5
✔ LifePoints 35

Afternoon Snack Six

a glass of carrot juice
3 or 4 spears of steamed asparagus on a bed of alfalfa sprouts with low-fat French dressing – all on a slice of pumpernickel bread
a small tub of low-fat fruit yogurt
✘ RiskPoints 9
✔ LifePoints 36

Afternoon Snack Seven

a glass of pineapple juice
a sandwich with Bean pâté, cos lettuce, cucumber and cress
a handful each of dried apricots and dates
✘ RiskPoints 10
✔ LifePoints 47

DINNERS

Dinner One

a starter of fresh mango
pineapple juice
followed by steamed couscous with chickpea and vegetable stew
a side dish of steamed, spiced spinach and baked squash
after which chopped dates topped with plain low-fat yogurt and a sprinkling of ground coriander
✘ RiskPoints 29
✔ LifePoints 71

Dinner Two
a starter of half a cantaloupe melon
vegetable juice cocktail
followed by lasagne made with TVP mince
a mixed side salad (no fish, meat or cheese) with low-fat Italian
dressing
after which matzos with Bean Pâté
✘ RiskPoints 29
✔ LifePoints 83

Dinner Three
a starter of fresh orange segments
orange juice
followed by steamed white rice with dhal, steamed and spiced
spinach, sweet potato and mixed vegetable pilau made with a
yeast extract sauté of spices
after which fresh lychees
✘ RiskPoints 28
✔ LifePoints 92

Dinner Four
a starter of fresh pineapple slices
orange juice
followed by a bowlful of chilli salsa (made with TVP mince)
served with ready-to-bake tortillas and spiced black beans
with a mixed side salad (no fish, meat or cheese) with low-fat
French dressing
after which banana bread
✘ RiskPoints 23
✔ LifePoints 61

Dinner Five
a starter of rice cakes spread with Bean Pâté
pineapple juice
followed by spaghetti in tomato and vegetable sauce
a side salad of chopped spring onions, parsley and beansprouts
with low-fat French dressing
after which half a cantaloupe melon
✘ RiskPoints 30
✔ LifePoints 57

Dinner Six

a starter of pasta and white bean soup with French roll
carrot juice
followed by a salad platter of mixed salad (no fish, meat or cheese) topped with steamed asparagus spears and low-fat thousand island dressing
matzos spread with Bean pâté
after which fresh watermelon
✘ RiskPoints 29
✔ LifePoints 79

Dinner Seven

a starter of banana milkshake made with skimmed milk and a banana puréed together
orange juice
followed by a three-bean salad made with green beans, kidney beans and blackeye beans tossed with chopped spring onion, low-fat French dressing and juice of 1 lemon
served over chicory greens (escarole or batavia)
with a small slice of tomato olive pizza, no cheese
after which a plate of fresh grapes, strawberries and nectarine slices
✘ RiskPoints 19
✔ LifePoints 99

PART FIVE: THE LIFEPOINTS SHOPPER'S GUIDE

When you first begin to construct your LifePoints larder you may feel you are performing more of a *de*construction. Certainly, some of the products that you give shelf space to at the moment will have to go to give room for the high-LifePoints foods you intend to introduce. Here are the steps we recommend.

Step One: begin the clear-out!

Shelf by shelf, pull everything out, wipe down the cupboard and gradually put things back, *but* put all the foods high in RiskPoints to one side. That means that the crisps, the creamed coconut, the tinned steak and kidney pudding and the half-eaten treacle tart get piled on to the kitchen table for the time being. Also, keep to one side those double-zero foods that lurk in every cupboard: the jar of instant coffee, the cans of fizzy drinks, the jams and that bottle of butterscotch topping. Get them all out!

Repeat this clear-out with your refrigerator. Pull everything out and wipe down the inside of your fridge. Now, gradually put back only those foods which are high in LifePoints, discarding any that are old and emptying all those anonymous plastic containers which have stood undisturbed for so long. Set high-RiskPoints and double-zero foods to one side.

Finally, tackle the freezer. This is more of a sorting job, putting the high-LifePoints foods into one freezer compartment and the high-RiskPoints foods in another.

Now decide whether you wish simply to discard the high-RiskPoints and double-zero food items you have cleared from your freezer, fridge and cupboards, or whether you are happy to pass them on to someone else. Alternatively, you might go through a period of 'grossing out' on bad food! This is not something we recommend but we know that some people will do it so we mention it here to show you all the options. What you need to end up with is a larder – freezer, fridge and cupboards – that is clear of the foods which will present a real obstacle to your LifePoints goals.

Look now to the foods which you have kept and do some fine-tuning.

Step Two: check the sell-by dates

Position your stock of food on the shelves with the oldest food in front, where you will use it first. If you have ever worked in a shop, you will understand this is simply 'stock rotation', and ensures that the minimum amount of food gets wasted. This same method of organization can be employed in the fridge and freezer, putting older foods to the front or top.

Step Three: check the quality of storage

For each food type:

- Check that your freezer holds the standard temperature of −18 °C (0 °F) with a reduced temperature of −23 to −25 °C (−5 to −10 °F) for the compartment used to freeze food from fresh.
- Buy a thermometer for your fridge if you haven't got one already. The recommended temperature is no higher than 5 °C (41 °F) to prevent loss of nutrients, food spoilage and possible food poisoning.
- Although it may seem the safest thing to keep eggs in the fridge, it isn't. Condensation can unplug tiny, porous holes in the shell, allowing dangerous bacteria to penetrate. Pull your eggs out of the fridge and store at room temperature in a pretty wire basket or china bowl.
- Collect those bottles of oil from your worktop and cupboards and put them into the fridge – similarly, any shelled nuts. The cold temperature will help to slow down the process of oxidation which turns them rancid.
- Expand the 'crisp' section of your fridge – that area near the bottom used to store fruits and vegetables. Vegetables lose around 70 per cent of their folic acid content within three days if they are stored in daylight, so the cool dark fridge is a perfect alternative.
- Make sure the food cupboards are cool and dark. If they are not, try moving the food to a cupboard that is, maybe one that is currently used for china or even household odds and ends. Specifically, root vegetables, fruits and any food item in a clear glass bottle or jar needs to be stored in a cool dark place.
- Make sure storage containers are airtight and preferably dark glass, metal or heavy-grade plastic. All dry produce, such as

beans, flours, rice, muesli, etc., will keep well in these conditions, but if you transfer it from its original packaging, it is worthwhile writing the use-by date on a small sticky label and pressing this on to the container.

- Herbs and spices, though often sold in clear glass jars, are best kept in airtight dark glass or earthenware containers. In years gone by, spices and herbs were kept in special cupboards, which were characteristically dark, dry and cool. Try to do the same for your herbs and spices – they will taste much better for it.

Now that you have completed the clear-out, you can begin to fill the gaps in your larder with high-LifePoints foods. Here are a few tips to help you get the most from your shopping routine.

ORGANIZING YOUR SHOPPING

Even the most organized people can get a bit frazzled when they go shopping. There is something about the pace at which we live, the crowds in every aisle and the abundance of produce that makes shopping a potentially chaotic and frenzied part of living. It is more than common for people to come home with items they don't really want or with a bill that is larger than they have budgeted for. Here are some steps that will help you keep your cool, your money and your LifePoints goals.

Step One: always make a shopping list!

Try to make it during a calm and quiet part of the day, rather than just moments before you are due to shop. Making a shopping list used to be commonplace a few decades ago; today, most people don't bother. This is a great pity, because it deprives you of that absolutely vital element of *control* over your shopping purchases. In fact, it cedes control to the shop or supermarket you visit. Beneath that clean, efficient and smiling exterior lurks an awesome selling machine geared up to induce you to buy, buy, buy. Everything in the modern supermarket, from layout to logo, sound to smell, taste to touch, is designed to make you purchase. You entered the store to buy a bag of sugar, you leave with a full trolley and an empty wallet. Why? Consider the tactics they employ against you:

- Lighting. Strategically placed lighting often exaggerates the succulence of even the most anaemic and unappetizing produce. The overall brightness of the store emphasizes the fresh, clean and efficient atmosphere.
- Sound and smell. Unpleasant, intrusive sound is kept to a minimum. Air conditioning or equipment noise is silenced by soothing mood music to relax you into a state of pliable consumption. The seductive aroma of baking bread stimulates impulse sales; test tastings of cheeses, wines and cooked meats are yet another weapon in the sales armoury.
- Colour and texture. Dark wood trim and decor conveys a rustic, traditional illusion – a strong appeal to the desire for a country kitchen packed with tasty, country produce.
- Layout. Products are displayed so as to maximize customer flow: the more you see, the more you will buy. Essential items are kept far apart to ensure that you wander all over the shop. Old stock is pushed to the front, the fresh, new goods put to the back of the shelf. While you wait interminably in the checkout queue – where did that time go that you were supposed to be saving? – your kids will pillage the choc bars placed there specifically to get their attention.

Of course, you can't really blame the supermarkets for wanting to sell their products as hard as they can. However, these tactics are clearly designed to benefit the shopkeeper – not you, the customer. This is why a well-organized shopping list is imperative if you are to save your own time, money and sanity. Unorganized shopping is extremely wasteful as you inevitably come home with unwanted items, only to find you forgot the one essential you needed most! Fortunately, today's technology can help you here. There are countless variations on the traditional shopping list, ranging from the wipe-clean slate on the kitchen wall, which can be easily updated, to the hand-held computer (such as the Newton), which can actually go shopping with you, add up all the prices, and save you money if the checkout operator incorrectly enters your purchases. Use whichever method you're happiest with. What is most important, however, is that you use some method to plan your shopping in an orderly and organized way. And once you have planned, don't surrender to impulse purchases! Compile your list in this order:

1 Fruit and vegetables: fresh, frozen, tinned or bottled.
2 Cereal and grain staples: such as pasta, flours, rice, couscous, bread.
3 Nuts and beans: dried, frozen, tinned, butters and spreads, etc.
4 Household requirements: such as toilet paper, soaps, toiletries.
5 Optional food extras: such as snacks, drinks, convenience foods.

Here is an example of how your list might look:

FRUIT AND VEG: FRESH
lettuce, spring onions, tomatoes, apples, bananas, mangos
Fruit and Veg: Frozen
spinach, cauliflower, peas, raspberries
Fruit and Veg: Tinned or Bottled
sweetcorn, chopped tomatoes, apple sauce, figs in light syrup
Cereal and Grain Staples:
lasagne, cannelloni, linguine, plain wholewheat flour, polenta, basmati rice, bulghur (cracked wheat)
Nuts and Beans: Dried
red lentils, split peas, butter beans
Nuts and Beans: Frozen
green beans
Nuts and Beans: Tinned
kidney beans, borlotti beans, chickpeas
Nuts and Beans: Butters, Spreads, etc.
tahini, peanut butter, tofu
Household Requirements:
shampoo, toothpaste, paper napkins, floor polish
Optional Food Extras:
pretzels, tonic water, Jimmy's birthday cake mix

Step two: double-check
Double-check your larder and amend your list if necessary to ensure your larder is stocked with the high-LifePoints essentials you will come to recognize. Here is our 'essentials' list as an example:

Fruit and Vegetables
1 lb of fruit per day per person, in season only
in season vegetables for salads
in season vegetables for soups and stir fries
Cereal and Grain Staples
plain wholewheat flour, couscous, wholegrain rice, polenta, pasta
– all sorts
Nuts and Beans
tahini paste, tofu, soya milk, red lentils, chickpeas, kidney beans
(dried and tinned), frozen or tinned green beans
Optional Food Extras
popcorn kernels

Step Three: go shopping!

Enter the shop and pick up a basket or trolley, according to how much money you intend to spend, and select your produce *in the order of your list.* Try not to waver from this rule, no matter how enticing the product you are faced with.

Tip: Buy only what you can store properly. It's no use spending good money on produce that will only go to waste or lose nutrients quickly once you have it home.

Tip: Plan your shopping route through a supermarket, shopping precinct or marketplace – again, in the order of your list – to make your expedition more efficient and successful.

Tip: Use small convenience shops with a specific product in mind, i.e. a missing tin of tomato paste, or you are more likely to buy on impulse and perhaps unwisely, i.e. snack or convenience foods that don't enhance your LifePoints goals.

TIPS FOR DEFENSIVE SHOPPING

Perform the Freshness Test

● **Smell**   All fresh food should have a fresh smell; there is nothing at all wrong or improper in holding a piece of fruit or a vegetable to your nose and smelling it. After all, you are not putting it up your nose and you will wash the food before using it anyway.

• **Skin check** Look for bruises, gashes, mould, bird pecks and splits when buying fresh fruit and veg and try to do this without adding any to the poor thing! Although we don't mind the odd bird peck – easy to cut them out – a split tomato or mouldy lemon is just about the worst item of shopping to unpack once you get home.

• **Stem and root check** Avoid buying broccoli, carrots, parsnips and the like that have begun to rot. A piece of broccoli may look wonderfully green on top but be brown and mushy at the stalk end. This indicates that it is many days since that broccoli was harvested and most of its nutrients will have long since departed. Similarly, root vegetables such as carrots can begin to rot where the greens used to be and it is easy to overlook this moist, brown area in favour of their orange-coloured appeal.

Check the use-by date

Old produce will have suffered severe nutritional decay. Shopkeepers often put older stock at the front of the display – it's called 'stock rotation' – so rearrange their display, and buy from the back.

Buy it only when you need it

With the advent of today's massive, out-of-town hypermarkets, the temptation for all of us is to do a 'big shop' once a week, every couple of weeks, or even once a month. While this may be an effective way of saving your shopping time, it can also lead to considerable overstocking of your larder with highly perishable food. All too often, this results either in the spoilage and discarding of significant quantities of fresh food or, even worse, in the consumption of food which is extremely stale. This is bad for two important reasons.

First, it can be the direct cause of food poisoning. Every year, about 1.5 million people suffer the effects of food poisoning, and at least 100 deaths are directly attributable to it. Second, it results in you eating food whose nutritional content has been substantially degraded. LifePoints figures for food in the Counter have been calculated for food eaten in a wholesome state; but if you're not eating good fresh food, then you simply can't expect the figures to give you an accurate reflection of your nutrient status.

So make it a rule to consume perishable food as quickly as possible after purchase, and for preference, buy your fresh food on a daily basis, from a good local store. It's also worth looking out for fruit and vegetables that are in season, and locally grown when possible. These are more likely to be fresh and therefore richer in nutrients than their well-travelled cousins. If this is not possible, select (in this order of preference) frozen, bottled, dried or tinned fruits and vegetables.

Go for whole food

Lean towards buying food which is as whole and unrefined as possible. In general, the more a foodstuff is processed, the greater the loss of natural nutrients. Wholewheat flour, brown rice, and wholegrain breads are some examples. Similarly, select nuts that are sold still in their shells. These stay fresh for longer and the fats they contain are less likely to be rancid.

FOOD POISONING – PROTECT AND SURVIVE!

1 Cook everything thoroughly. If you still eat meat, it's worth investing in a meat thermometer. Beef should be cooked to an internal temperature of 60 °C or above for rare, 70 °C for medium and 77 °C for well done. Lamb and pork need to be cooked to an internal temperature of 77 °C.

2 Never eat raw eggs in any form (e.g. mayonnaise) – always make sure they're thoroughly cooked.

3 Although it may seem to be the safest thing to keep eggs in the refrigerator, it isn't. Condensation can unplug tiny, porous holes in the shell, allowing dangerous bacteria to penetrate. And the lowered temperature of the yolk means it needs even longer cooking.

4 Don't buy tinned goods which are damaged – no matter how good a bargain they appear to be. Small cracks in the lining inside the cans affect the contents, which will certainly affect the delicate vitamins and other nutrients and may even cause the food itself to turn bad.

5 Be particularly careful if you use a microwave oven. The evidence suggests that you shouldn't rely on it to

---

kill off bacteria in your food. Always follow the recommended standing times.

6 Never reheat food more than once. Make sure it's not underheated.

7 Be certain that frozen food is thoroughly defrosted before cooking.

8 Be sure all kitchen towels, sponges, surfaces, food equipment and cutting boards are kept clean. When you're preparing a meal, it's also prudent to wash utensils and worktops between stages – don't use the same knife or chopping board for raw meat, cooked food and fresh vegetables without washing it between times. Meat is a major cause of food poisoning – keep it well away from other foods.

9 Store raw and cooked foods separately. Never leave leftover canned food in its tin.

10 Put all rubbish and scraps of food straight into the waste bin – and always keep the lid securely down, so that flies can't get in and germs can't get out.

11 Cut down on the quantity of food you cook. This reduces the amount of leftovers in your diet, which are a major source of food poisoning.

12 And above all – don't take chances. If your food smells off, throw it away.

PART SIX: THE LIFEPOINTS KITCHEN

The way in which you prepare your food can either safeguard and unlock those precious LifePoints nutrients or wipe them out entirely. Here, we'd like to share with you some secrets, hints and tips we've personally found to be effective not only in delivering maximum nutritional value from our food, but also for doing it in a speedy, easy and tasty way!

Cooking a food changes starches, proteins and some vitamins into accessible forms for us to absorb, as well as releasing nutrients in some foods which are otherwise bound in, like the amino acid tryptophan in cornmeal. And for some foods, proper cooking is absolutely necessary in order to destroy harmful substances. For example, a recent outbreak of the deadly haemolytic uraemic syndrome, whose symptoms include bloody diarrhoea, intense abdominal pain, stroke-like bleeding in the brain and culminate in irreversible damage to the intestines and kidneys, was caused by the victims eating undercooked hamburger meat. Nevertheless, cooking is generally harmful to the nutrients in food, but there are certain ways of minimizing the inevitable nutrient loss which takes place during the cooking process:

- Pressure cooking is one of the best ways to reduce nutrient loss in appropriate foods. Invest in a non-aluminium pressure cooker, which, because of the shortened cooking times, will also reduce energy consumption and therefore the size of your fuel bills.
- After pressure cooking, steaming and microwave cooking are the next healthiest options. Buying a steamer is obviously a lot cheaper than buying a microwave oven! Further down the list are (most valuable first): boiling, grilling, stir frying (at high temperature where the fat seals in the nutrients), sautéing and, finally, deep frying.
- If you cook with fat, don't let it become so hot that it starts to smoke. At this temperature the essential fatty acid linoleic acid is destroyed immediately.
- Fats which have been used for cooking once must be

discarded since the linoleic acid and many other vitamins will have been lost.

- If you boil food, do so for the minimum amount of time and then use the water for stock afterwards. The fragile water-soluble vitamins, as well as some minerals, leach into cooking water (which is why soups are so nutritious).

- Don't add bicarbonate of soda to cooking water, even if you see it recommended in recipes (for example, for cooking pulses). It destroys valuable B vitamins.

- Chop and prepare food barely seconds before you cook it – remember that vitamin C is destroyed once cells are damaged in vegetables – and for the same reason try not to chop them too finely. Scrubbing vegetables is better than peeling them.

- Once you have prepared them, steam or cook the vegetables in ready boiling water straightaway.

- Use pans with close-fitting lids and avoid using copper pans, which encourage oxidation and vitamin C loss.

- Once food is cooked, eat it straight away. Keeping it warm will only result in further nutrient loss, which is why eating out too frequently may be less than healthy for you. (See 'Escaping from the Kitchen', page 111.)

- For a quick, no-fuss and nutritious lunchtime snack at work, cook a giant pot of soup on Sunday evening and freeze it in lunch-sized servings. Take one out of the freezer every morning and reheat it at work (for more soup recipes, see *LifePoints Cookbook*).

- Most beans and vegetables can be cooked and then marinated all day or overnight for a really exquisite flavour (there are some really great marinades in *LifePoints Cookbook*). The beauty of marinating is that the food may be stored, covered, in the fridge and used as snacks, salads or lunches for the next 3 or 4 days. All are high in LifePoints and, if you make the marinade oil-free, low in RiskPoints too.

- Prepare a grain or lentil loaf (see *LifePoints Cookbook*) and slice leftovers into sandwiches and salads during the next 2 or 3 days.

- Add zero-RiskPoints, high-LifePoints foods freely to enhance your enjoyment of each meal and snack. Most people find the quantity of food listed in each menu more than ample but adding LifePoints-only foods will ensure you don't go hungry and that, if you feel a snack coming on, you have plenty of options from which to choose. The listings on page 114 give you plenty of examples.

Finally, if you lead a hectic lifestyle, and consider that you don't have time for some of the advice given above, think again. The life you lead is totally dependent on a good nutritional support system – without which, you're just running on empty. And you can only do that for so long.

ESSENTIAL TECHNIQUES

Cooking beans
Most beans double in bulk once they are cooked.

- Measure the beans into a mixing bowl and pick them over to remove any stones or unwanted pieces of bean.
- Cover the beans with cold water and wash them very well by swirling your hand through them and exerting a scrubbing motion. Pour the water away and repeat this process three times, or until the water is clear. Drain the beans.
- Cover the beans with fresh water and leave them to soak overnight or all day while you are at work. Soaking the beans helps to prevent the flatulence that some people suffer from after eating beans.
- Drain the beans and throw the water away. Rinse them under running water, drain them, then tip the beans into an iron pot and cover them with water. Bring them to the boil, reduce the heat and simmer with the pan partially covered for 1 to 3 hours, depending on the type of bean you are cooking. The beans must remain covered in water and they must cook until they are easily squashed between your tongue and the top of your mouth. If they are undercooked you will get a stomach ache.
- Alternatively, some beans may be pressure cooked. Cover the beans with water, seal the cooker and bring up to pressure. Cook at pressure for 20 to 40 minutes, depending on the type of bean you are cooking. (Please refer to the leaflet accompanying your pressure cooker.)
- In both methods, adding a strip of kombu (seaweed) to the water will help to soften the beans.

- Red lentils and split peas do not require soaking or pressure cooking. They do require washing. Red lentils are especially quick to cook and are therefore very useful for a quick, nutritious meal.

Chickpeas	25 minutes in the pressure cooker; 3 hours in the pot.
Kidney beans	25 minutes in the pressure cooker; 1½ hours in the pot.
Butter beans	20 minutes in the pressure cooker; 1½ hours in the pot.
Soybeans	30 minutes in the pressure cooker; at least 3 hours in the pot.
Blackeye beans	20 minutes in the pressure cooker; 1 hour in the pot.
Lentils and split peas	40 minutes–1 hour in the pressure cooker; 1 hour in the pot.

Cooking rice

Rice is *not* a difficult food to prepare! The instructions that follow are the very easiest you are ever likely to come across, and you really can't go far wrong.

- Put some rice into a pan. There is no need to measure anything, just be aware that it will more or less double in volume by the time it is cooked.
- Pour in lots of water. This is the most important stage: the rice must be very well cleaned, and this has to be done by hand, so, immersing both hands, give the rice a good scrub, passing it through your fingers and rubbing vigorously. You will see husks and other debris come to the surface, and the rice will make the water quite milky. Drain the dirty water, add fresh water and repeat the scrubbing movement. Do this for three changes of water; after the third change, the rice will no longer make the water milky.

- Drain all the water out. With your fingers, roughly level the rice in the pan. Now pour in fresh, cold water, to twice the volume of the rice. Therefore, if the rice fills the pan to a depth of one inch, pour in enough water to fill the pan to two inches.
- There is no need to add anything else, such as salt, to the water. Good quality brown rice has enough natural flavour not to need any enhancements, and condiments such as soy sauce can be added at the time of serving if required.
- Cover the pan. Place it on a medium to high heat, and bring to the boil. When it starts to boil, reduce the heat as much as possible to maintain a fairly low simmer. Do not remove the cover.
- Cook the rice for about 45 minutes. This time will vary slightly according to the exact type of rice, your cooker, etc. At this time, take a peek at the rice and push it open with a wooden spoon, to see if there's any remaining water at the bottom of the pan. The rice is perfectly finished if the very bottom layer of grains turn slightly yellow and start to adhere to the pan. This, incidentally, is considered by macrobiotic cooks (who know a thing or two about preparing rice) to be the very finest, most health-giving of all rice. If you are preparing the rice to coincide with the cooking of various other foods, you can turn the heat off completely and, keeping the pan covered, simply let the rice steam itself for the last five minutes or so of its cooking. This will keep it nice and warm and give you a few minutes of extra time to attend to the other foods.

Sprouting beans and seeds

Any seed is capable of being sprouted, but the most flavoursome are legumes such as peas, beans, fenugreek, alfalfa and clover, and vegetables such as parsley, amaranth, celery and lettuce. All that is required is air, moisture and a jar – so there is no reason why you should not soon have your own crop of this invigoratingly healthy and versatile food! Here's how to sprout this very popular alfalfa, though the method will suit any seed:

- Use a container with some sort of drainage, such as a colander, strainer, mesh tray, or even a flower pot with a cloth net over the hole. A jar with a piece of cheesecloth or muslin held in place around the top with a rubber band is perhaps the simplest and most effective. The size of the jar depends on how many seeds you are sprouting, but it should hold at least half a litre.

- Seeds can be bought from health food stores, where they are usually labelled 'organic', and some supermarkets. Do not buy seeds from agricultural merchants – they may well be contaminated with seed dressing chemicals which might be fatal if consumed. Use only the clean, whole ones and throw out the rest.

- For every decilitre the jar holds, use between two and three tablespoons of seeds. First they must be soaked in four times their own volume of water, ideally filtered or mineral water, until their bulk is doubled. This normally takes about eight hours, or overnight. After this time, pour off the water. It contains a lot of the seeds' goodness and so should be used in cooking if possible.

- The sprout container should be kept in darkness – just throw a tea towel over the jar. The seeds must be rinsed two or three times a day through the muslin mesh of the jar. Make sure you drain them thoroughly each time by turning the container upside down, or the sprouts will rot.

- Throw away any seeds that have not sprouted after two days. The rest will be ready to eat after four or five days. On the last day they can be put into the light, but only for a few hours or they will become bitter.

- Most sprouts will need a final rinsing and draining before being put in the fridge in a covered container for storage. Some varieties, however, have loose husks which need to be removed. Place these sprouts in a large bowl of water and agitate until the husks float to the top, then you can skim them off.

Grain or vegetable sprouts do not require cooking, but bean or pea sprouts should be simmered quickly to make them easier to digest, following the times given in the table below:

Mung bean sprouts	3 minutes
Lentil bean sprouts	10–15 minutes
Peas	5 minutes
Chickpeas	8 minutes
Fenugreek	3 minutes
Soya beans	soak for two hours, rinsing frequently, and then cook for 10–15 minutes

Vegetable sprouts are good in salads and sandwiches, or as a garnish for any dish. Grain sprouts can be used in bread: just mix into the dough before baking. Bean sprouts can be steamed with other vegetables or stir fried for a couple of minutes. Sprouted alfalfa seeds are a rich source of vitamin C and certain B group vitamins, and can be added as an interesting garnish to salads, or can be used to accompany almost any sandwich filling.

THE LIFEPOINTS SAUTÉ

Sautéing is one of the most enticing cooking methods because, in addition to producing those lovely appetizing aromas, it also creates sensual sizzling sounds that start us all salivating with anticipation! However, even though sautéing adds less fat to food than deep frying or pan frying, it still adds enough fat to your diet to blow a hole through your day's RiskPoints limit. The problem we were faced with, therefore, was how to replace this attractive method of food preparation. It took us a lot of tastings to discover the best alternative, but we think you'll agree that the following technique – the LifePoints Sauté, as we call it – really does preserve all the lusciousness of a traditional sauté, without the fat! Try it once or twice and you'll quickly get the hang of it – so you can use it in all the recipes you see which use sautéing as part of their technique.

- First, dissolve 1–2 teaspoons of yeast extract in 60–90ml (2–3 fl. oz) water and bring this to a quick simmer in a frying pan or saucepan over a medium heat. Add the onions, garlic or whatever is to be sautéed and stir for 2–5 minutes (or the recommended time, if you're following a recipe). The aroma is enticing, the sizzle is there and the flavour and texture created are excellent. In addition, the yeast extract adds valuable LifePoints to your total.

- Once you have become familiar with the LifePoints Sauté, adjust it by trying other liquids, such as tomato sauce, in place of the yeast extract dilution.

FLAVOUR TO THE MAX!

You're not going to succeed in reducing the amount of fat you consume if all you do is you pine for the taste and texture that fat gives food. Instead, we strongly urge you to start to experiment with other techniques and dishes. Start cooking with fresh herbs, spices, garlic, onion, scallions, flavoured vinegars, and high-quality mustard to boost your food's flavour – there's a whole world of flavour out there, just waiting for you to explore! Try using herbs and spices to add gorgeous new flavour combinations to food while it's being steamed (a very good way to preserve nutrients and protect natural juices). And if you really want to enjoy the taste of oil, buy strongly flavoured ones – such as walnut or basil olive oil – and use a pastry brush to thinly apply it to food after the cooking process. This really makes a little oil go a long way!

Also, actively experiment with new sauces and dressings. Fruits, vegetables, and legumes can all be used to create purées, relishes, coulis and compotes. Relishes – known as salsa in Mexico, chutneys in India, and sambals in Indonesia and Malaysia – can be hot or cold, chunky or smooth. Add them to rice, pasta, steamed vegetables or meats.

- **Herbs** Dried herbs are best added during cooking so that their essential oils distribute through the food. If fresh, they are often best added towards the end of cooking or just before serving so as not to lose the delicate flavours fresh herbs produce. For instance, fresh basil may be added to a tomato sauce almost as a garnish when you serve it, yet it will still impart that exquisite aroma and flavour to the whole dish. Experiment in your own cooking and even try growing a pot of basil, parsley or thyme on your windowsill or terrace so that you have these otherwise expensive condiments to hand.

• **Spices** These are often best added at the sauté stage so that their essential oils distribute well but also 'mature' during the rest of the cooking process. Some spices, such as black pepper, are especially good added at this stage. Others, such as the curry collection of spices, are often best added just before the end of cooking so that their flavours do not deteriorate. Again, experiment with a light hand to begin with, until you get to know the results you may expect.

Warming Spice and Herb Blend

This is a robust blend which we love – it may be used alone or in combination with Mild and Fresh Spice Blend in savoury dishes. The ingredients may be adjusted to suit your taste.

Makes 140g (5 oz)
Serves 4
Preparation time: 15 minutes

5 spring onions, finely chopped
3 cloves garlic, finely chopped
1 tablespoon fresh ginger, grated
1–2 fresh hot chillies, finely chopped
2 tablespoons fresh basil, chopped
1 teaspoon freshly ground cardamom
1 teaspoon freshly ground black pepper
¼ teaspoon ground nutmeg

Blend all the ingredients and add to the dish during the sauté stage.

Mild and Fresh Spice Blend

This mixture can be used to flavour soups, stews and other dishes; adjust it to suit your taste. This amount is for one dish.

Makes 3–4 tablespoons
Preparation time: 10 minutes

1 tablespoon caraway seeds
3 cloves garlic, crushed
2 teaspoons fresh ginger, grated
1 teaspoon freshly ground black pepper
1 teaspoon ground coriander
½ teaspoon salt
¼ teaspoon ground allspice

Grind all the ingredients in a mortar and pestle until the caraway seeds are slightly crushed. Stir into the dish, either during the sauté stage or shortly before serving, and adjust to taste.

Garam Masala

This spice mixture may be changed to suit your tastes. Use a mortar and pestle, a hand-turned peppermill or an electric grinder, such as a coffee grinder, to grind your spices. It is best, and noticeably different in flavour and aroma, to use whole spices – grinding them only when you need them. We all have a need for little short cuts now and again, however, so simply store any surplus ground spices in a labelled, airtight jar in a dark cupboard. This amount is for one dish.

Makes 2–3 tablespoons
Preparation time: 5 minutes

2 teaspoons freshly ground coriander
1 teaspoon freshly ground black pepper
1 teaspoon freshly ground cumin
½ teaspoon freshly crushed cardamom
½ teaspoon freshly ground cloves
½ teaspoon freshly ground cinnamon

If you can, grind these spices individually, measure them, then mix them. Alternatively, if you know that you will cook with garam masala within the next 7–10 days, prepare a double or triple recipe, blend the spices and simply use half or one-third of it today. Garam masala is traditionally used in Indian cooking.

THE LIFEPOINTS RECIPE UPGRADE

When you adopt the LifePoints lifestyle, your old and much-loved favourite recipes need not necessarily become things of the past. You can often transform these old favourites into high-LifePoints, low-RiskPoints dishes by performing one or two simple amendments. Here is a ten-point recipe-upgrade pro-gramme we think will work with most of your past glories:

1 Does it include pastry? Substitute with New Pastry (*LifePoints Cookbook*).

2 Does it include a sauté stage? Use the LifePoints Sauté (page 97).

3 Does it include eggs? If it includes them for texture and colour, use mashed tofu and turmeric. If the eggs are used for binding purposes, use a little agar powder, breadcrumbs or a tablespoon of rice flakes. If they are for raising purposes, use egg substitute plus an agent such as baking powder, as appropriate.

4 Does it include fish? Try using Quorn instead, which is available from most supermarkets.

5 Does it include fatty meat? Use textured vegetable protein (TVP) or a product such as VegeMince instead. This is now widely available, both in supermarkets and health food shops, and is available in mince and chunk form. It is also available in plain, beef or chicken flavours. As you can see from the listings (see meat substitute in the Legumes section), TVP is very high in LifePoints and definitely counts as one of our value-added foods.

6 Does it include milk? Use skimmed milk or soya milk, or substitute another liquid such as fruit juice or vegetable stock.

7 Does it include cream? Usually low-fat plain yogurt will do instead.

8 Does it include cheese? First, reduce the amount asked for by three-quarters, adding rice flakes or lentils to make up for the

texture and binding qualities. Second, try eliminating it entirely and use tofu or nutritional yeast flakes instead (available from health food shops). Remember that a robust cheese flavour can often be produced by using a small amount of very strongly flavoured cheese, such as Parmesan.

9 Does it include sugar? Try using a small amount of blackstrap molasses instead. Whilst adding its own definite flavour, it also adds a few LifePoints, something sugar is sadly lacking.

10 Is it deep fried? Sorry, find a new favourite! Deep frying, in our language, is the same as deep trouble.

MAKEOVERS FOR LEFTOVERS

Leftovers are a fact of life for most of us – they just happen, even to the most organized cook. The most vital aspect about using leftovers effectively is to use them *as soon as possible* (see our remarks about food hygiene, page 88). And we firmly draw the line at 'recycling' food once it has been put on someone's plate. (Peter's first holiday job as a teenager was working at an expensive restaurant where, amongst other horrors, he had to scrape the unused salad cream from diners' plates back into the container for re-use – it put him off eating at restaurants for years!) That being said, here are some nifty tips for maximizing the value from your food purchases:

Fruit

There are times when you over-purchase and then realize you can't eat it all before it will start to go off, or times when you arrive home with a bag full of squashed peaches because the bus driver braked too hard and sent you and your sack hurtling into another passenger! For those times, and many others you can probably think of, it is useful to have an easy way of salvaging the situation and the damaged fruit.

Fresh but otherwise unattractive fruit can be mixed with soya or skimmed milk in a blender to make a milkshake. Add a little ground spice of your choice (try coriander, nutmeg or allspice) to give it some zing and serve chilled, if possible. Here is our favourite, the Banana NutriShake from *LifePoints Cookbook*:

Banana NutriShake

Most milkshakes are far too high in RiskPoints. This one isn't – because we use soya milk, and because we don't add anything apart from bananas and a hint of spice. Choose a good brand of soya milk, which includes extra calcium and vitamin B12. Try adjusting the flavouring to your taste – we've found ¼–½ teaspoon of vanilla extract combines gorgeously with the bananas, or alternatively you could try the same amount of rum extract. None of these flavourings is going to affect the RiskPoints – so, hey, go wild!

Serves 4
Preparation time: 10 minutes
✔ *LifePoints per serving: 17*
✘ *RiskPoints per serving: 4*

1 l (2 pints) soya milk, chilled
very ripe bananas, peeled
1 teaspoon ground nutmeg

Purée the soya milk, bananas and nutmeg together in a blender. Divide the mixture between four large tumblers (preferably pre-chilled), stir briskly and serve at once.

Fresh peelings, cores and sundry pieces of fruits such as apples, pears, rhubarb, plums and berries can be turned into a yummy fruit butter. Wash the fruit and turn it into a large enamel saucepan with a tiny amount of water added to the mixture. Cover and place over a low flame, stirring frequently, until the mixture is very soft and the separate fruits have lost their shape. Add a little brown sugar and some ground spice to taste and cook for a further 5 minutes. Then rub the mixture through a sieve, discard the rough pulp and eat the rest today! Children and adults alike are fond of this surprise fruit butter. And it is especially wonderful because it uses whatever you have to hand, so no two batches are alike. We like it warmed, but it is delicious cold as well.

Bruised or dented pears and apples may be peeled and sliced then left in the fridge to marinate in a mixture of wine or fruit juice and fresh herbs or spices. Try a cup of red wine, gently warmed in a pot with whole cloves and a small piece of cinnamon, then poured over the fruit slices. Make sure the fruit is covered, then leave the dish to cool before chilling it in the fridge until you are ready to serve it.

Bananas that look too ripe for your children's tastes can be diced into a tahini and banana sandwich instead – before they ever get to see the brown speckles. Of course, to some people the speckled sort is the perfect sort, but even then it's worth making this sandwich – it's delicious!

Vegetables

You bought the broccoli on Friday and by noon on Saturday you realize it is not going to fit into your ever-changing plans. Do you helplessly watch as it turns yellow? Never! Steam it right now until just tender and still bright green then remove it from the heat and leave it to cool. An hour later, when you fancy a little snack, arrange the broccoli on a plate with a little low-fat French dressing or some spicy salsa. Instant! Alternatively, you could add the steamed broccoli to a salad for extra depth and robustness. Or again, you could marinate a collection of vegetables. Once you start to think inventively and creatively, there's really no limit to what can be done. Here, for example, is our Vegetable Marinade from *LifePoints Cookbook*:

Vegetable Marinade

Serves 8
Preparation time: 45 minutes plus cooling and chilling time
✔ *LifePoints per serving: 15*
✘ *RiskPoints per serving: 2*

for the marinade:
285ml (10 fl. oz) cider vinegar
juice of 2 lemons
whole cloves
whole peppercorns
1 teaspoon caraway seed
140ml (5 fl. oz) apple juice

bayleaves
small pieces of stick cinnamon
425ml (15 fl. oz) water

the vegetables:
225g (8 oz) carrots, scrubbed and thinly sliced
450g (1 lb) green beans (fresh, tinned or frozen)
small red pepper, chopped
small green pepper, chopped
small onions, thinly sliced
medium cauliflower, trimmed and cut into florets
450g (1 lb) broccoli, trimmed and cut into florets

Gently heat all the marinade ingredients together in a large enamel saucepan while you prepare the vegetables. Do not bring to the boil yet. Add all the vegetables to the marinade, stir well and bring to a low boil. Cover the pan and simmer gently for 15 minutes. Remove the pan from the heat and allow the mixture to cool, stirring the mixture once or twice as it does so. Serve immediately or keep chilled in the fridge for 3 or 4 days. This marinade improves in flavour for being chilled. It is excellent as a lunch, picnic or light evening meal.

More ideas: steam some root vegetables with the broccoli – parsnips, potatoes and carrots, for instance – then mash the whole lot together with some skimmed milk and pepper for an exquisite, colourful mash that your children especially will love.

Take all the clean peelings, tops and tails, outer leaves and unpresentable veg and put them into a giant pot along with a handful each of barley, oats and fresh herbs. Bring to the boil, then cover and simmer gently for about one hour. Leave to cool, then strain this broth and measure into soup-sized portions. Keep one in the fridge and freeze the rest for your later convenience. Here is our recipe for Vegetable Stock from *Life-Points Cookbook*:

Vegetable Stock

Makes approximately 2 l (4 pints)
Serves 8
Preparation time: 2 hours plus cooling time
✔ *LifePoints per serving: 7*
✘ *RiskPoints per serving: 1*

55g (2 oz) barley or scotch broth mixture
3 l (6 pints) water
450–675g (1–1½ lbs) root vegetables or parts (i.e. peels, tops
and tails, chunks), washed
225–450g (½–1 lb) greens or outside leaves (i.e. unsightly
leaves, green parts of cauliflower, leaves of celery, coarse lettuce
leaves, cabbage hearts), washed
large onions, coarsely chopped and including the skins
bulb garlic, coarsely chopped and including the skins
bayleaf
any chopped fresh herb or bouquet garni
1 teaspoon whole peppercorns
1 teaspoon whole cloves
a piece of cinnamon stick

Measure the barley and water into a large saucepan and place
over a high heat. Bring the mixture to a boil, stirring frequently.
Add the remaining ingredients and stir well. Cover the pan,
reduce the heat and leave to simmer for 45 to 60 minutes, stirring
just occasionally and skimming any froth from the surface.

Leave the mixture to cool, then strain the stock through a
colander or sieve and discard the vegetable matter. Use the stock
at once or measure it into portions for freezing and later use.

Certain classic or traditional dishes are actually based on leftovers, so don't feel shy about conserving your scraps. Here are
two you are sure to recognize:

Bubble 'n' Squeak

This is made of precooked vegetables that are roughly chopped the next morning and sautéed (LifePoints Sauté, please! See page 97) together over a medium heat. We like ours with freshly ground black pepper and tomato ketchup.

Vegetable Patties

Precooked vegetables can be finely chopped and mixed with spices, rolled oats or cooked rice and a little water. Once they are shaped into patties, they can be grilled or sautéed in a LifePoints Sauté mixture (see page 97) and served as part of a warming breakfast or lunch.

Even more ideas: add vegetable pieces to a sauce before you purée it to improve its texture and add depth to its flavour.

Lightly steam the vegetable pieces, then douse them in a spicy tomato sauce, cover the dish and leave to cool. Suddenly you have a scrumptious vegetable marinade that can be served as a side dish, chutney or dressing for a main dish.

Cereals

Leftover rice, millet, couscous and pasta may all be put to excellent use, providing you use them quickly. Here are some inspirations for you:

- Most salads are enhanced when a *little* of any of these cereal products is tossed in with the vegetable mixture.
- A bean or vegetable soup is also enhanced when small amounts of rice or pasta are stirred in towards the end of cooking.
- Rice, millet and couscous – as well as odds and ends of rolled oats, rice flakes or puffed grain breakfast cereals – are easily converted into a useful grain loaf. Simply stir them together with a packaged vegetable sausage or burger dry mix, some strong spices and dried herbs, and a blend of water and tomato paste until the mixture has a firm but moist texture. Press it into a loaf tin and bake in a hot oven for about 30 minutes. Now pour a little tomato sauce over

the loaf and bake a further 10 minutes. Remove from the oven, leave to cool in the pan for about 5 minutes, then turn it on to a plate to slice and serve. This is delicious hot, with rice, a collection of steamed or baked vegetables and a light sauce. We thinly slice a cooled loaf to make sandwiches or fill pitta breads.

- Speaking of breads – if you make your own bread, you can add a little cooked rice or millet to the dough. Work it well in, so that the grains are held by the dough, then bake in the usual way.

Nuts and Beans

Yes, even these can be used. Here are a few ideas:

- Dried beans often lurk in the cupboard in cellophane bags, each one containing precisely twelve beans. What good is that? Get them all out, pour them together into a bowl and cover them in water. Later today or tomorrow, drain them, rinse them and add them to a soup or stew. Or, if you have a pressure cooker, cook them, cool them and add them to a salad.
- Cooked beans can also be mashed together with spices and sautéed onions and garlic to make a sandwich spread or dip.

Red Bean Paste

This is a recipe that is wonderfully close to refried beans, of Mexican cuisine fame.

Serves 4
Preparation time: 40 minutes plus cooling and chilling time
✔ *LifePoints per serving: 9*
✘ *RiskPoints per serving: 0*

115g (4 oz) dried kidney or pinto beans, washed and soaked overnight
1 teaspoon yeast extract
3 tablespoons water
5 cloves garlic, finely chopped
2 small onions, finely chopped
1 teaspoon chilli powder

1 tablespoon soy sauce
2 tablespoons cider vinegar
285–425ml (10–15 fl. oz) vegetable stock or water

Drain and rinse the beans and pressure cook them for 25 minutes. Drain them immediately. Dissolve the yeast extract in the water, pour into a large pan and place over a medium to high flame. When the mixture begins to bubble, add the garlic and onion and sauté for two minutes, stirring often. Add the chilli powder and stir a further minute.

Add the soy sauce, vinegar and the cooked beans to the sauté and mash them slightly as you gradually add the stock. Aim for a thick, rough paste. Serve hot (see Mexican Tostadas in the *LifePoints Cookbook*) or allow to cool and chill in its serving dish. Useful as a dip, pâté or sandwich spread.

Bean Pâté

This is another all-time favourite of ours, which tastes as if it's very high in RiskPoints but in fact has none.

Serves 8
Preparation time: 45 minutes plus cooling and chilling time
✔ *LifePoints per serving: 11*
✘ *RiskPoints per serving: 0*

225g (8 oz) dried red lentils, washed and drained
1 teaspoon yeast extract
570ml (1 pint) water
1 teaspoon turmeric
85g (3 oz) rice flakes
1 teaspoon freshly ground black pepper or ½–1 teaspoon chilli powder
2 teaspoons ground ginger

Turn the lentils into a saucepan. Dissolve the yeast extract in the water, pour over the lentils, place on a medium to high flame and bring to a soft boil. Cover the pan, reduce the heat and simmer for 30 minutes, stirring occasionally.

Add the turmeric, rice flakes, pepper and ginger and cook over a low flame for a further 5–10 minutes. Remove from the heat and spoon into a serving dish. Press the pâté well down into the dish. Allow the pâté to cool, then cover and chill before serving. This looks wonderful garnished with parsley or lemon slices.

This recipe can be altered to make use of precooked beans of any sort. Simply cook the beans, mixed in with the remaining ingredients, and press into a ramekin or pudding bowl before leaving to cool.

Shelled nuts should be used as soon as possible. Any leftovers may be ground and added to bread, cake or biscuit recipes. Alternatively, they may be stirred together with leftover grains, vegetables and beans to make burgers or a loaf. Add a little tomato sauce to the mix then sauté, grill or bake in the usual way.

Precooked beans may be mixed together and cooked in a marinade. Kept chilled, this marinade can provide snacks and lunches for three to five days.

Five-Bean Salad

Serves 12
Preparation time: 30 minutes plus cooling and chilling time
✔ LifePoints per serving: 18
✘ RiskPoints per serving: 6

450g (1 lb) cooked kidney beans
450g (1 lb) cooked green beans
450g (1 lb) cooked chickpeas
450g (1 lb) cooked butter beans
450g (1 lb) cooked borlotti or pinto beans
5 spring onions, thinly sliced
1 eating apple, grated
5 cloves garlic, crushed
1 tablespoon fresh ginger, grated
1 teaspoon brown sugar
2 teaspoons freshly ground black pepper
5 whole cloves
1 piece of stick cinnamon
285ml (10 fl. oz) cider vinegar
juice of 4 lemons

Measure all the ingredients, except the lemon juice, into a glass or enamel saucepan and stir well. Place the pan over a medium heat, cover and bring to a slow boil. Reduce the heat and simmer, covered, for 10 minutes.

Leave the pan covered and remove from the heat. Allow to cool, then stir in the lemon juice and turn the salad into a separate dish to chill in the refrigerator. This salad improves as it cools and may be kept, chilled, for two to three days.

Grind leftover nuts and mix some ground spices in with them. Freshly ground black pepper and cumin seed is a wonderful savoury mixture; ground allspice and coriander is a delectable sweet mixture. Sprinkle the ground nuts over a salad or bowl of fresh fruit or lightly roast the mixture in a frying pan (without oil) for 3 or 4 minutes over a medium flame. Serve the same day on to lightly steamed greens or freshly steamed rice or couscous.

ESCAPING FROM THE KITCHEN

Even the most ardent home cook wants to escape from the kitchen at some time or other and sit down to a meal cooked by someone else. And for other people whose jobs involve an element of business entertainment, restaurant dining can become an occupational hazard. It can be very difficult to find high-LifePoints, low-RiskPoints food in some restaurants, so here are some valuable tips which work for us, and which will help you get maximum LifePoints and minimum RiskPoints from your meal out.

Know the no-no's

There are some foods and dishes that seem, on a first glance at the menu, to be healthy, but are secretly a storehouse for RiskPoints. Here's our shortlist:

Potato: sautéed potatoes and potato salads are probably best avoided, as are mashed potatoes, which are made with lots of milk and butter. Baked potato is a good food that is often spoiled by being doused in butter. Order baked or steamed potatoes without the fat.

Ratatouille: this delicious dish is made with large quantities of olive oil. Perhaps there is a vegetable soup or pickle on the menu instead?

Risotto: a wonderful rice dish but, again, made with large quantities of olive oil. How about a simple mixture of steamed rice and wild rice instead?

Pastries: sorry, most are rather high in RiskPoints. Would a toasted crumpet or bagel do instead?

Nuts: watch for these high-RiskPoints foods in muesli, nut butters, savoury snack mixes, snack bars and biscuits.

Cheese: for some reason, professional chefs find it hard to be sparing when cooking with cheese, so try not to order a dish that contains it. Pizza parlours usually have one or two options already on the menu – we've always enjoyed tomato sauce with olive and fresh basil topping. The fresh basil is good by itself, too. If you don't see it on the menu, ask for it.

Aubergine: this food is a sponge for oils and fats. Try to avoid it.

Soufflé: somehow this dish is always a combination of milk, cheese, cream and eggs. Whoa!

Cream of . . . : anything that says 'cream of' is a bit of a no-no (see cream of mushroom soup at 59 RiskPoints, for example), though you can, at home, whip up a low-RiskPoints 'cream of' alternative.

Sauces and dressings: These must be taken carefully and with a light hand. There are many low-fat dressings and sauces available, so ask for them. Otherwise, a squeeze of fresh lemon will enhance most salads and steamed vegetables and *a few drops* of a sesame or walnut oil will give deep flavour. Again, ask!

Plan ahead

If you can, learn the type of restaurant and style of food it serves before you go out. This isn't always possible and, in any case, you should think ahead and plan what you will order if it is on the menu. Here are some dishes we suggest you bear in mind as likely to be low or moderate in RiskPoints:

Starters

- In-season melon or fresh mango
- Any fruit juice
- Gazpacho or minestrone soup
- Steamed asparagus spears with low-fat dressing

- Mixed salad (no fish, meat or cheese) with low-fat dressing.

NOTE: By all means, have a starter. It is easy to find one with few or no RiskPoints and you'll feel better for it.

Main Course
- Couscous with chickpea and vegetable stew
- Pasta with simple tomato sauce, no cheese
- Sweet pepper stuffed with rice, vegetable and tomato mixture, no cheese
- Steamed rice and dhal with spinach and potato (**NOTE:** This meal will vary according to the chef; go for one not floating in ghee).
- Pizza with tomato sauce, olives and fresh basil, no cheese.

Desserts
- Fruit salad, from fresh or dried fruits
- Iced yogurt
- Sorbet
- Baked apple
- Fresh figs, lychees, mango, melon, strawberries, raspberries or poached pears.

NOTE: No cream or ice cream, please!

Just Say No!
Whatever you do, don't be bullied by restaurant staff or your friends, colleagues or companions into eating what you don't want. Most restaurants are aware of a growing interest in healthy eating and will happily cater for your needs. We happen to think, however, that going with plenty of information and ideas like those we have just suggested will make your meal out a more satisfying and pleasant one. Bon appetit!

The following foods contain NO RiskPoints but a useful number of LifePoints.

THE LIFEPOINTS TOP TEN OF EVERYTHING

Position	Food	RiskPoints ✗	LifePoints ✔
1.	GrapeNuts (Standard serving 30g)	0	25
2.	Corn Flakes, Kellogg's (Standard serving 30g)	0	17
3.	Old potatoes, baked, flesh and skin (1 medium potato 156g)	0	15
4.	Carrot juice (1 cup 246g)	0	14
5.	Beet greens, boiled (1 cup 144g)	0	12
6.	Yeast extract, fortified with vitamin B12 (1 teaspoon 5g)	0	11
7.	Nori, dried, raw (1 sheet 10g)	0	11
8.	Turnip tops, boiled (½ cup chopped 72g)	0	11
9.	Chicory greens, raw (½ cup chopped 90g)	0	10
10.	Cabbage, chinese (pak-choi), boiled (1 cup shredded 170g)	0	10

LIFEPOINTS TOP TEN FRUITS

Position	Food	RiskPoints ✗	LifePoints ✔
1.	Apricot, dehydrated (low-moisture), sulphured, uncooked (½ cup 60g)	0	8
2.	Pineapple juice, canned, with added vitamin C (1 cup 250g)	0	8
3.	Prune juice, canned (1 cup 256g)	0	8
4.	Apricot, dried, sulphured, uncooked (½ cup halves 65g)	0	7
5.	Orange juice, canned (1 cup 249g)	0	7
6.	Pineapple juice, canned (1 cup 250g)	0	7
7.	Acerola juice (1 fl. oz 30g)	0	6
8.	Apricot, dehydrated (low-moisture), sulphured, stewed (½ cup 124g)	0	6
9.	Currant, zante dried (½ cup 72g)	0	6
10.	Orange, raw (fruit 131g)	0	6

LifePoints Top Ten Cereals

Position	Food	RiskPoints ✗	LifePoints ✔
1.	GrapeNuts (Standard serving 30g)	0	25
2.	Corn Flakes, Kellogg's (Standard serving 30g)	0	17
3.	Spaghetti, canned – Asda Healthy Choice (lower in sugar and salt) (½ can 205g)	0	10
4.	Macaroni, plain, cooked (1 cup 115g)	0	7
5.	Macaroni, vegetable, cooked (1 cup 134g)	0	5
6.	Barley, pearled, cooked (½ cup 79g)	0	4
7.	Bulghur, cooked (½ cup 91g)	0	4
8.	Wild rice, cooked (½ cup 82g)	0	4
9.	Couscous, cooked (½ cup 90g)	0	3
10.	Rice, white, long-grain regular, cooked (½ cup 79g)	0	3

LIFEPOINTS TOP TEN VEGETABLES

Position	Food	RiskPoints ✗	LifePoints ✔
1.	Old potatoes, baked, flesh and skin (1 medium potato 156g)	0	15
2.	Carrot juice (1 cup 246g)	0	14
3.	Beet greens, boiled (1 cup 144g)	0	12
4.	Yeast extract, fortified with vitamin B12 (1 teaspoon 5g)	0	11
5.	Nori, dried, raw (1 sheet 10g)	0	11
6.	Turnip tops, boiled (½ cup chopped 72g)	0	11
7.	Chicory greens, raw (½ cup chopped 90g)	0	10
8.	Cabbage, chinese (pak-choi) boiled (1 cup shredded 170g)	0	10
9.	Sweet potato, canned (½ cup 127g)	0	9
10.	Vegetable juice cocktail (1 cup 242g)	0	9

LIFEPOINTS TOP TEN LEGUMES AND NUTS

Position	Food	RiskPoints ✗	LifePoints ✔
1.	Pinto beans, canned (½ cup 120g)	0	9
2.	Pea, split, boiled (½ cup 98g)	0	8
3.	Pea with carrots, canned (½ cup 128g)	0	7
4.	Aduki beans, boiled (½ cup 115g)	0	7
5.	Pea with carrots, frozen, boiled (½ cup 80g)	0	6
6.	Bean sprouts and mung beans stir fried (½ cup 62g)	0	5
7.	Lentil, sprouted, raw (½ cup 38g)	0	5
8.	Mange-tout, raw (½ cup 72g)	0	5
9.	Lentil, red, canned in tomato sauce (1 average serving 115g)	0	4
10.	Green beans/French beans, boiled (½ cup 62g)	0	3

PART SEVEN: LIFEPOINTS POWER FOODS

───────

When you switch to a high-LifePoints diet, you know that you're changing to a way of eating that's going to provide you with the most nutritional boost from your food. As you know, the whole philosophy of the LifePoints system is to provide you with a powerful and easy way to prioritize your diet – putting most emphasis on those foods (with high LifePoints and low Risk-Points) which are going to deliver the maximum health-enhancing nutrition, with a minimum amount of unwholesome components. We know from the responses of many readers that a great many people want and expect even more from their diets – they would like to be able to 'let their food be their medicine', and choose their day's food intake on the basis that food can and should be able to prevent or ameliorate many of the disease states which currently afflict millions of people in Western societies. Well, simply changing to a high-LifePoints, low-RiskPoints way of eating is a very good beginning indeed. And for many people that alone will be enough to achieve significant health benefits. But if you want to go further – and 'fine tune' your diet by choosing specific foods to combat or prevent certain disease states – LifePoints Power Foods can help. This is not intended to replace the advice of a qualified health practitioner, but it *can* help you to take the LifePoints concept a stage further, by differentiating between foodstuffs on the basis of their physiological effects. In the following pages, you'll find the remarkable health benefits associated, by scientific studies, with the consumption of specific foods. These foods – LifePoints Power Foods – can, together with the LifePoints system, form the bedrock of the world's healthiest way of eating.

LIFEPOINTS POWER FOODS: ACNE

The vast majority of people have suffered from acne at some point during their lives. Teenagers who suffer from it are not unusual – one study estimates that 90 per cent of teenagers are afflicted by it at some time. Acne often seems to develop at about the time that most people's bodies start to mature and increase their production of certain types of sex hormones. And some of us will go to extraordinary lengths to cure this teenage curse. When a raider in a balaclava and dark glasses held up a Scarborough chemist's shop at gunpoint, it wasn't cash he was after. Handing the startled assistant a bag, he demanded: 'Fill it up with spot cream!'[13] As you might expect, the market for acne treatments is thriving – over £30 million is spent on anti-acne skin products in Great Britain alone.

As the level of sex hormones increases in the body, little glands under the surface of the skin, called sebaceous glands, start to increase their production of sebum. Sebum is an oily substance that is used to lubricate the skin, and it normally moves freely to the surface of the skin. Problems develop, however, when its progress is blocked by hard plugs of skin called keratin. As the blockage increases in size, it may show up as a whitehead, developing into a blackhead when it becomes coloured by skin pigmentation. In the meantime, sebum production continues unabated, and sebum may leak into the surrounding skin, causing inflammation. If bacteria are attracted to the developing mass of sebum, they may then produce free fatty acids, which will inflame the skin further. The skin becomes irritated, pus and cysts may form, and scar tissues develop.

Now, although acne has traditionally been reserved for spotty teenagers, more and more adult women, even those who have never had skin problems before, seem to be suffering from so-called execu-rash. In mature women, it seems as if the stress of today's lifestyle can cause their bodies to overproduce male hormones, or androgens. Produced by the adrenal glands in response to stress, androgens stimulate oil glands in the face, shoulders, chest and back. Excess oil then plugs their pores, and bingo! Acne develops.

Many drugs have been used to try to control acne. Some chemicals will make the horny layer of your skin soften and peel away; these substances are termed keratolytics. The aim is to remove the plugs of keratin, so allowing the sebum to drain freely. Some of these substances can be effective – for some people.

Products sometimes contain anti-bacterial substances, but since acne is not actually caused by bacteria, although they may play a rôle in its continuance, it's not certain how effective these products will be. In general, drugs that are sold over the counter in chemists' shops may have some use in treating mild cases of acne, but more severe cases will require treatment by a medical dermatologist.

In recent years, it has become received wisdom amongst conventional medics that diet and acne are not related. That's because a number of experiments have failed to pinpoint any one ingredient of the diet either as a universal trigger or as a cure for acne. But we already know that acne is caused by a number of factors – not just chocolate pudding. And new evidence from all over the world is starting to indicate that, while food may not be the only cause, it may well be part of the problem.

When scientists studied clear-skinned and blemish-free Eskimos and Japanese who switched to eating a Western diet, they found cases of acne suddenly appearing. And the Zulus of South Africa have always had a spotless skin as well, until they were moved from their tribal villages to the cities, where they ate Western food and developed acne.

Essential fatty acids

Essential fatty acids (EFAs) are called 'essential' because your body can't manufacture them itself, and it relies on you to eat a good diet to obtain its supplies. According to research published in the *Journal of the American Academy of Dermatology*, acne sufferers have been found to have a deficiency of the EFA linoleic acid in their skin – this could well be due to too much hydrogenated fat in the diet. So you may be able to help your body fight acne by replacing the hydrogenated fats in your diet, which can actually cause a deficiency, with oils which are rich in linoleic acids, such as sunflower, soybean, corn or safflower oil.

Vitamin A

Research proves that people with very severe acne often have low levels of vitamin A in their blood. It has long been known that this vitamin is essential for skin maintenance. As the cells in the skin renew themselves rapidly, vitamin A, with its important growth properties, is particularly vital for this organ, the largest in the human body. In fact, several of the commercial drugs currently available for acne treatment are vitamin A-based. Plants contain a form of vitamin A known as carotene, found in carrots, which can be converted in the human body to vitamin A. Good, natural sources are carrots themselves, green leafy vegetables such as spinach and broccoli, and fruits which have a characteristic yellow colour, such as peaches, mangos and apricots. A diet which is rich in these foodstuffs will naturally supply all your vitamin A needs. Retinol supplements should only be used under professional advice, because there is evidence that adverse effects, including birth defects, may be caused by doses of 25,000 IUs or higher.

Chromium

It has been estimated that as much as 90 per cent of the population may have a deficiency of this trace element. Chromium works in the body to convert blood sugar into insulin, and researchers have found that the more insulin the body uses to process sugars following meals, the more chromium the body needs. And, indeed, it has been found that people with unstable levels of glucose in their blood are more likely to develop severe acne – one researcher has even called acne 'skin diabetes'. In one experiment, researchers found that patients with unstable levels of blood glucose also experienced severe acne. When they were given two teaspoons daily of high-chromium yeast containing 400 micrograms of chromium, their improvement was rapid.[14] To increase your chromium intake, eat plenty of brewers' yeast and molasses.

Hormones

The male hormone testosterone stimulates production of the sebaceous glands and is triggered in times of stress. This may be the reason why more and more older women are developing acne. As they are put under increasing stress from both work and family, their testosterone levels shoot up, with acne as one of the results. Since many animal foods contain hormones and hormone-like substances, it might be a good idea to avoid these foods if you fall into this category. Beauticians have also reported that women who eat a lot of meat are more likely to have body hair, because of the steroids the meat contains.[15]

Iodine

Try avoiding iodine-containing foods for a while and see if your skin condition improves. It seems that even minute amounts of iodine may lead to skin problems in sensitive people because any excess that the body cannot absorb is excreted through the pores, aggravating a condition such as acne. So try avoiding foods containing significant amounts of iodine, such as kelp, seaweed, asparagus, liver, milk, wheat and particularly cough mixtures and tonics.

Selenium

For a long time, scientists thought that selenium was simply a toxic substance which had no dietary use at all. But recent research suggests that very small amounts of selenium (200 micrograms, which is the same as 0.2 milligrams) taken twice daily for six to twelve weeks, in combination with vitamins A and E, can reduce the severity of persistent acne.[16] Selenium is naturally found in broccoli, cabbage, onions and whole-grain products.

Zinc

Experiments have found that both oral and skin application of zinc has brought positive results in people with acne. In one experiment, 58 per cent of sufferers reported dramatic improvement when treated with zinc. Millions of people are zinc-deficient in the West, probably due to their consumption of over-refined foods. The best natural sources of zinc include wholegrain products, brewers' yeast and pumpkin seeds.

Allergies

In experiments it has been shown that about 10 per cent of acne sufferers can reduce their symptoms by finding, and eliminating from their diet, a food to which they're allergic. The most common foods to produce this reaction are almonds, malt, cheese, mustard, red pepper and wheaten flour.

LifePoints Power Foods: Arthritis and Rheumatism

Arthritis is a specific term describing inflammation of the joints; rheumatism is used more broadly and describes all aches and pains in the muscles, bones or joints. In this sense, we have all suffered from rheumatism at some time. Rheumatoid arthritis is therefore inflammation and pain of the joints *and* the surrounding tissues. There are, in fact, some 100 different types of arthritis, including:

- Reiter's Syndrome, an acute form often accompanied by eye inflammation and more frequently found in young men.
- Ankylosing Spondylitis is a chronic complaint, affecting the spine, pelvic joints, and sometimes the heart and eyes. It causes pain, fatigue and depression which can last for years.
- Systemic Lupus Erythematosus is much more common in women and is characterized by skin rashes and joint inflammation.
- Gout involves swelling and severe pain, normally in the big toe. It has long been known to be aggravated by diet, especially foods rich in purine, which produces uric acid.

Why do people get arthritis?

Many different causes have been suggested, including stress, allergy, food and environmental pollution, malnutrition, hormonal imbalance and digestive inadequacy. Another cause is that our body can mistakenly attack itself in trying to fight off foreign bacteria that closely resemble our own tissue. This is called an auto-immune response. Relevant to all of these, there is ever increasing evidence that diet has a very important rôle to play in the onset and control of these degenerative disorders.

- People who significantly change the bacteria colonizing their gut often experience relief from rheumatic symptoms.[17] A change of diet, such as described below, as well as a course of colonic irrigations followed by the use of acidophillus supplements will begin to improve your internal hygiene.
- One interesting study of rheumatoid arthritis involved a week of fasting followed by three weeks of a non-animal products diet. At the end of this time, 60 per cent said they felt better, with 'less pain and increased functional ability'.[18] The diet was essentially similar to the sort of high-LifePoints diet you would consume when choosing foods from the first four food groups only (i.e. the compulsory ones!).
- In another study, rheumatoid arthritis sufferers given a fat-free (i.e. low in RiskPoints) diet for seven weeks reported a

complete absence of symptoms.[19] When animal and vegetable fats were returned to their diets, their symptoms returned. So try restricting your RiskPoints intake to 100 or so, and make sure all of the food chosen only contains non-animal fats.

- More specifically, meat and dairy products contain the fatty acid arachidonic acid, which promotes the inflammation that is felt in rheumatism and arthritis when it converts to inflammatory prostaglandin and leukotrienes. Replace animal fats with foods high in polyunsaturates and the omega-3 fatty acids (found in flaxseed oil supplements) to experience less pain.

- Vitamin A is necessary for the body to fight infection, a key in many rheumatoid cases. To make sure you get enough of this vitamin, eat plenty of yellow, orange and green fruits and vegetables such as spinach, carrots, papaya, pumpkin, sweet potato, watercress and parsley.

- If you are taking drugs for a rheumatic disease, it is probable that you are lacking in vitamin B complex. This is found in whole grains and brewers' yeast.

- Vitamin C helps to thin the synovial fluid in your joints, which leads to improved mobility. Arthritics particularly benefit from taking vitamin C because the aspirin they take to reduce pain and inflammation depletes the body of vitamin C. Fresh citrus fruit, blackcurrants, green peppers and cauliflower are all excellent sources.

- Vitamins C and E and the mineral selenium are all antioxidants; oxidation is a process in which nutrients in the body are broken down before the body can use them. Selenium also reduces the production of prostaglandins and leukotrienes, both of which cause inflammation. Whole grains, vegetable oils and nuts are rich in vitamin E, and usually good sources of selenium.

- Avoid purine-rich foods such as organ meats, peas and beans if you suffer from gout.

- A New England horticulturalist has developed a theory that solanum alkaloids, found in members of the nightshade family of plants, could cause arthritis in some people. The nightshade family includes deadly nightshade, aubergine, red and green pepper, potatoes, tomatoes and tobacco. A group of

3000 sufferers cut this family of foods from their diet and experienced reduced aches, pains and disfigurement.[20]

- People with arthritis sometimes have an enzyme deficiency in their small intestine which means they are unable to absorb gluten, a protein found in wheat flour. In fact, maps of areas where gluten-high cereals are eaten correspond to those areas with the highest incidence of rheumatoid arthritis.[21] And countries where rice or corn is the staple grain show a much lower rate of the rheumatic diseases than those whose staple grain is wheat. Reduce your consumption of gluten by substituting rice cakes and oatmeal or corn bread for wheat bread and cake.

- Food intolerance creates symptoms which include headaches, fatigue, depression, constipation and, in some people, rheumatic pain and stiffness. If you suspect you are intolerant of a particular food, eliminate it from your diet completely. Here's how:

  1 Stop eating the food in any form for eight weeks. If that food *is* causing you problems, you will probably crave it for several days and generally feel terrible.

  2 Were you to eat the suspect food at this craving stage and feel very much better, then you are undoubtedly intolerant of it. This may seem paradoxical – but food intolerance closely resembles addiction at this stage.

  3 After approximately ten days your craving will diminish.

  4 After 14 to 18 days, eat a little of the suspect food. If your symptoms return, your suspicions are confirmed and the food has caused you problems.

  5 Some people may eat very small amounts of this food infrequently with no ill effect after avoiding it for 2 to 3 months. Others experience a complete return of symptoms if they ever eat the food again.

- Yucca is a folk medicine which has been used for more than 1000 years in America. In a study into its effects, 60 per cent of rheumatoid arthritis and osteoarthritis patients experienced an improvement in their symptoms of swelling, pain and stiffness.[22] Yucca is available in supplement form.

LIFEPOINTS POWER FOODS: CANCER

The causes of cancer are multifarious. Genetic, dietary, occupational and psychological factors all play an important part. In fact, it is unusual to be able to pinpoint a single cause of cancer and say, 'If it weren't for this, I would not have cancer'. Rather, cancer seems to form out of a lifestyle in which some detrimental factors are occupational, some psychological, some dietary, and so on.

Various observations have been made in recent decades:

- The number of cancer cases has risen dramatically in recent years until nearly half of all cancers are suffered by just one-fifth of the world's population – those who live in industrialized countries.[23] And of course, industrialized populations have to cope with more stress, pollution and degenerative diseases than non-industrialized populations.

- People who are generally viewed as 'nice' people – slow to anger, compliant, unassertive and overly cooperative and patient – seem more likely to succumb to cancer. Those who have an aggressive manner or a 'fighting spirit' seem more likely to combat or even conquer it.[24]

- Carcinogens (cancer-producing substances) are found in many areas of life, from work to leisure to the home. Of these, many are self-administered; some knowingly, as in cigarettes and radiation; others unknowingly, as in various pollutants whose effects may be suspected but are not yet fully known.

- When eminent scientists Richard Doll and Richard Peto assembled all the evidence they could linking the occurrence of human cancers to specific identifiable causes, they estimated that 'diet' was the greatest single risk factor – responsible for approximately 35 per cent of all deaths due to cancer. 'Tobacco' came second (30 per cent).[25]

The influence of diet in the development of cancer is probably the most predictable and the simplest to control. Here are the components of your diet which you can manipulate to reduce your risk of developing cancer.

Fat – cut it out!

Generally, there is a much lower cancer rate in countries where the average diet is made up of less than 30 per cent of calories from fats. In the UK and America – where cases of cancer are much higher – the average fat intake is 42 per cent of calories from fats.[26] A wide range of cancers seem to be particularly associated with a high-fat diet, including breast, ovarian and colorectal cancers. Colorectal cancers are especially common in countries with a Western-style diet, rich in meat and fatty foods.[27] In countries where a traditional low-fat, high-fibre diet is still followed, these cancers are noticeably rare. A good LifePoints diet will, of course, provide you with many good sources of fibre whilst keeping your fat consumption under tight control.

Omega-3 fatty acids are being studied to see whether they can reduce the risk of breast cancer in some women.[28] It seems possible, based on information available thus far, that these fatty acids may prevent or reverse an abnormal metabolism of hormones which signal an increased risk of cancer. Omega-3 fatty acids are present in flaxseed oil.

Fibre foods

Fibre is the cornerstone of many healthy-eating regimes, and a diet naturally high in fibre can almost certainly lower your risk of cancer of the colon.[29] It is thought to protect you from cancer by adding bulk to your diet – thereby preventing concentration of carcinogens as the digestive process proceeds. It may also help to eliminate potentially carcinogenic substances from the body quickly by speeding the transit of food through your digestive tract.

Vitamin A foods

A deficiency of this vitamin can contribute to the development of cancer in some people. It is available in two basic forms: retinol and carotene. Retinol is the form which your body makes and stores in fatty tissue round your eyes, liver and heart. When necessary, your body releases small, precisely controlled amounts of retinol into your circulation. Any excess is stored away, so if too much vitamin A in the form of retinol is taken, toxicity can occur. If you are taking a vitamin supplement, check the label to see what form of vitamin A is supplied. Retinol is found in flesh foods, especially liver, eggs, milk and cheese.

Beta-carotene is the form of vitamin A available in plant foods, and your body converts this form of vitamin A into retinol as and when your body requires it. Although large amounts of beta-carotene may cause your skin to take on an orange colour, this is temporary and not harmful – beta-carotene does not create toxicity in the same way that retinol can. Natural beta-carotene (not supplements) almost certainly has cancer-preventive properties.[30] In particular, it is thought to protect against cancers of the lungs, bladder, larynx and colon.[31]

Most researchers believe that beta-carotene is better than retinol for the purpose of protection from cancer. It is unlikely to cause toxicity, is a powerful antioxidant, is taken in and used according to the body's needs and comes in a 'package' including 'secondary plant constituents' – non-nutritive compounds that seem to inhibit the onset and growth of cancers and which may be vital to beta-carotene's anti-cancer action.

To obtain beta-carotene, eat any of the fruits and vegetables with a deep, bright green, yellow or orange colouring. Look for carrots, pumpkin, squash, spinach and broccoli, cantaloupe, sweet potatoes and papaya. Eat these foods raw, fresh and organically grown if possible.

Vitamin C foods

This vitamin helps to minimize the effects of pollutants and carcinogens (cancer-causing substances) in your food and environment.

- Vitamin C seems to block the formation of nitrosamines. Nitrates and nitrites are added to foods to give colour, flavour and to act as preservatives (E249–E252). During digestion these substances are converted by the human body into nitrosamines, which are known to be powerful cancer-causing chemicals (they are particularly associated with cancers of the stomach and oesophagus). The good news is that if a vitamin C-rich food is taken at the same time as foods containing nitrates or nitrites the production of nitrosamines is greatly reduced. Dr Helmut Bartsch of the International Agency for Research of Cancer in Lyons, France, discovered that regular doses of vitamin C (100mg three times per day) can dramatically reduce nitrosamine production.[32]
- Also, try to avoid foods which are high in nitrates and nitrites.

129

These include tinned, smoked and cured meats and fish, sausages, luncheon meats, bacon, pickled foods and some cheeses. In addition, tap water may contain these compounds, especially in farming areas where fertilizers containing nitrates are used on the land. Drink imported bottled water instead, and check the label for nitrate/nitrite levels.

- Mutagens are carcinogenic substances that can alter a cell's genetic make-up. They are readily formed when meat or fish is cooked to turn brown – for instance, when frying a burger or roasting a chicken. Although a high vitamin C intake may have a protective effect, you should reduce the amount of browned food you eat *and* increase your consumption of this vitamin.

- Another carcinogen, benzopyrene, is produced when meat is charcoal-grilled. Benzopyrene is also present in cigarette smoke; a 1 lb steak contains as much benzopyrene as the smoke of nearly 300 cigarettes. Avoid meats cooked in this way and, if you have been in the habit of eating them, greatly increase your vitamin C intake.

- Women with abnormal cervical smear results often have low amounts of vitamin C in their body.[33] This may shed new light on the underlying damage caused by smoking, because it has long been established that women who smoke have higher levels of cervical cancer. Smoking impairs the absorption of vitamin C but smoking also requires that you take more vitamin C to minimize the effects of it as a pollutant. If you do smoke, stop now! And greatly increase your intake of vitamin C-rich foods, such as citrus fruits, green peppers, broccoli, tomatoes, potatoes, cantaloupe and alfalfa sprouts.

Vitamin E foods

Vitamin E is another nutrient that provides protection against many of the damaging pollutants in the environment. It does this mainly by preserving oxygen in the blood, thus improving cellular strength and health. Of particular importance is vitamin E's ability to prevent the formation of free radicals, as well as its protective influence on vitamin A and C and the B group of vitamins. So, while vitamin E may not be in the 'front line' in your fight against cancer, it is essential to have a sufficiency of this vitamin in order to sustain improvements in your health.

- Vitamin E is destroyed by chlorine in your drinking water and by rancid oils; it may be rendered useless if oestrogen is also taken.
- Vitamin E is available in cold-pressed vegetable oils, nuts, seeds and soybeans.

Selenium foods

This trace mineral is essential to health, though only required in minute quantities. In America, the National Research Council has recommended a daily intake of 50–200mcg of selenium for adults (a microgram is one-thousandth of a milligram, so 200mcg equals 0.2mg). However, one authority – Gerhard Schrauzer, PhD, of the University of California – says that 250–300mcg can protect against most cancers, and that most people consume only about 100mcg daily.[34] But note that at higher doses, selenium can be toxic to the human body. Although it is not certain at precisely what level selenium begins to cause adverse effects, it has been found that doses of 900mcg (0.9mg) per day can make hair and nails fall out and can affect the nervous system.[35]

Selenium works best in conjunction with vitamin E, since both are antioxidants and can increase the production of antibodies by up to thirty times,[36] thereby greatly enhancing your immune response. Together they help to detoxify your body and prevent the formation of free radicals. Selenium is naturally present in the soil, and the quantities available in our food relate to soil levels of selenium where the food was grown. A study of selenium included a map of the soil distribution of selenium across the United States. This was then compared with a map detailing the national cancer rates. It was found that those areas with high levels of cancer corresponded with places of low levels of selenium in the soil. For instance, Ohio was shown to have the highest incidence of cancer and the lowest levels of selenium; South Dakota had the highest levels of selenium and the lowest rate of cancer.[37]

A study undertaken at the University of Tampere, Finland, involved taking blood samples from 21,172 Finnish men. The samples were then frozen. Eleven years after the samples had been taken, 143 men had contracted lung cancer. The researchers found that the men who eventually developed lung cancer had less selenium in their blood than those who did not. Overall, it was found that people with the lowest selenium levels were 3.3 times more likely to develop lung cancer than those with high levels. The researchers said their results were 'in accord with other studies which strongly suggest that poor selenium nutrition is a highly significant risk factor for lung cancer'.[38]

In Germany, a study conducted at the University of Bonn has shown that selenium can protect against the harmful effects of ultraviolet radiation. Blood selenium levels were examined in 101 patients with malignant melanoma (a lethal form of skin cancer) and compared to a control group of healthy people. The skin cancer patients showed a significantly lower level of selenium, and the researchers concluded that their results 'strongly suggest that sub-optimal selenium nutrition preceded the onset of the disease and may even have contributed to its genesis'.[39]

Selenium is naturally found in broccoli, cabbage, onions and wholegrain products.

Vitamin B Complex foods

Any form of stress, whether physical or mental, increases your need for the B vitamins. For instance, infection, pregnancy, the oestrogen pill, many drugs and the consumption of processed foods, coffee, sugar and alcohol all deplete your supply of this group of vitamins. The B's are vital for metabolism, the health of your nerves, skin and liver. While not in the 'front line' in the fight against cancer, the B group make other vitamins, such as A and E, much more effective in the work that they do.

- A high B intake is helpful in preventing cirrhosis of the liver; cirrhotic livers are 60 per cent more likely to become cancerous than healthy livers.[40]
- Foods richest in the B group are brewers' yeast and whole grains.

RiskPoints

Cancer seems to be more common in obese people, especially those who are more than 40 per cent over their ideal weight.[41] Following a low-RiskPoints diet (see *LifePoints Diet*) will help you to slim down and stay there!

Probiotics

It is possible to replace the harmful bacteria which flourish in your gut with immunity-enhancing bacteria called probiotics. A diet rich in refined foods, meat and fat seems to increase your likelihood of cancer because the various by-products of digestion create bacteria which are more likely to be converted into carcinogens. The addition of a probiotic such as *Lactobacillus acidophilus* inhibits this type of conversion and colonizes the gut. This alters the ratio of 'friendly' to 'unfriendly' bacteria and improves your health in several ways. The 'unfriendly' bacteria thrive after a course of antibiotics and after years of poor diet. The 'friendly' lactobacilli seem to enhance your immune function, prevent nitrites being converted to nitrosamines and convert nitrosamines back into non-carcinogenic substances.[42]

Lactobacillus acidophilus is just one of the friendly bacteria called probiotics; others are *L. bulgaricus, L. casei* and Bifido-bacteria. The lactobacilli are found in cultured dairy products such as yogurt.

Seaweed

Fewer women develop breast cancer in Japan than in either the US or the UK. The Japanese regularly include seaweed in their diet and some researchers now believe this has a major protective action against breast cancer.[43] Seaweed is thought to bind pollutants, inhibit the formation of carcinogens in the gut, reduce cholesterol and perform as an antioxidant. It also adds essential trace minerals to your diet.

Seaweed is a delicious and versatile food. Eat any of the common varieties several times each week.

Cabbage

Cruciferous vegetables include cabbage, broccoli, cauliflower, Brussels sprouts and kale. These foods contain what are called 'secondary plant constituents', non-nutritive compounds that seem to inhibit the onset and growth of cancers.[44] These compounds (i.e. indoles, phenols, flavones) are present in many plant foods but are particularly abundant in cruciferous vegetables. They are not available in supplement form.

Eat a serving of cruciferous vegetables three times per week, raw or cooked.

LIFEPOINTS POWER FOODS: CHOLESTEROL

Because it happens so slowly, you don't notice it. No one can *feel* their cholesterol level as it builds up, and even when an artery becomes more than half-blocked by the fatty, cholesterol-rich sludge known as 'atheroma', you still may not be aware of any warning signs to tell you that something is badly wrong. In fact, an artery usually has to be more than 75 per cent blocked before blood flow is seriously impeded. But by this stage, time is definitely running out. Our bodies depend on the normal flow of blood through minute capillaries, larger arteries (which transport oxygen-rich blood away from the heart) and veins (which carry blood back to the heart again) to nourish all our organs and body tissues. If this remarkable system, consisting of thousands of kilometres of blood vessels, is stopped for more than a few minutes, the heart will be damaged to such a great extent that it may be irreversibly stopped. So you see, with such a complex and awesome circulatory system, when something happens to interrupt or diminish your blood flow, the situation can become very serious, very quickly.

You will probably be shocked to learn that the very first clear, clinical account of someone having a heart attack was only written down in 1912. Until then, it seems that heart attacks were so rare they just weren't written about or recorded. Today, of course, heart disease is the commonest cause of death in the Western world. This means that heart disease is an *epidemic of the twentieth century*. It means that over the past 100 years, some-thing has happened to make a once rare and unusual form of death so common that by the age of 65 one man out of every five has had a heart attack and, of those, one in ten has died. Although two-thirds of heart attacks happen to men, this still means that in the United States, for example, about 400,000 women have a heart attack every year. But how do we go about lowering our cholesterol levels? There are several good ways. First and foremost, make sure that you are eating a low RiskPoints diet. This not only ensures that your total fat intake is healthily low, but it also makes certain that you are not obtaining too much of your energy from saturated forms of fat, which can make your cholesterol level skyrocket. In addition, there are further dietary steps you can take:

Soluble fibre

There can hardly be a person alive who hasn't heard of the benefits of eating a diet rich in fibre. But not everyone knows that there are two types of fibre – insoluble and soluble. Insoluble fibre is found in all plant foods, wheat bran being a major source. Insoluble fibre is highly effective for combating constipation, increasing stool weight, and preventing things like haemorrhoids and diverticular diseases. But it won't help reduce your cholesterol level.

Certain forms of soluble fibre, on the other hand, also have an effect on lowering raised serum lipids (fats in your blood). When a group of 18 healthy volunteers agreed to add either 23g of wheat bran or one 15g oat fibre tablet to their usual diet, the researchers found that the oat fibre was much more effective than wheat bran at lowering total cholesterol. 'The oat fibre tablet also proved easier to take and caused fewer side-effects,' reported the scientists.[45]

Now there are only relatively few foodstuffs which contain significant amounts of this special, cholesterol-lowering soluble fibre. Here they are:

Oats

It was observed at least as long ago as 1963 that oats could have a cholesterol-lowering effect. However, it is only in recent years that, as part of the quest for the answer to coronary heart disease, scientists have again re-examined this humble and inexpensive product. Today, many experiments have shown that oat bran can and does act to significantly lower blood cholesterol.

A group of twenty men with high blood cholesterol were admitted to hospital so their diets could be accurately measured for 21 days. Some were fed a 'control' diet (with no oat bran) and others were fed exactly the same diet but with added oat bran. After just three weeks, the men receiving oat bran supplementation had lowered their serum cholesterol concentrations by 19 per cent and had slashed their LDL concentrations by 23 per cent.[46]

Evidence shows that the average range of total cholesterol reduction on a low-fat diet with oat bran is in the region of 10–25 per cent. Of course, it depends to some extent on how high your cholesterol is to begin with. But a diet which includes about 100g of oat bran and lasts for at least three weeks (the longer the better) should show a useful improvement.

Oats are a natural substance which have been eaten for thousands of years, so any adverse reactions should be known by now. There may be a softening of your stools, which shouldn't be objectionable (it might be a welcome change!). You may have more wind, which should calm down after a short time. It is possible that if you are taking more than 50g per day some bloating or abdominal pain could occur, in which case you should reduce your intake and consult your doctor. As with all new diets, it would be advisable to consult your doctor prior to adding this amount of oat bran to your daily diet, so that your personal medical history can be taken into consideration. Perhaps the only real disadvantage is that it simply seems *too* easy. If you can achieve a useful reduction in blood cholesterol simply by adding oat bran to your normal food you may not take further steps to improve the rest of your diet. This would be a mistake. As Dr Basil Rifkind, Chief of Lipid Metabolism and Atherogenesis at the National Heart Lung and Blood Institute in Bethesda, says: 'It would be wrong for people to start consuming oat bran and forgetting about everything else. The main thing you want to do is increase complex carbohydrates in the diet and reduce the amount of fat you consume.'[47]

Corn bran

Corn bran (not as widely available as oat bran) may also be able to lower cholesterol. Researchers at Georgetown University Hospital found that when people ate raw corn bran their serum cholesterol was lowered by 20 per cent and triglycerides by 31 per cent. They gave about 40g daily to seven people suffering from hypercholesterolaemia, and, to make it palatable, flavoured it with garlic powder, black pepper and celery seed, and sprinkled it over tomato juice or soup. Apparently there were no serious side-effects.

Niacin

It has been known for some time that niacin – also called vitamin B3 – can lower cholesterol levels if taken in large amounts. Niacin is naturally found in foods such as yeast, milk, eggs, green vegetables and cereal grains, and your daily requirement of it comes to something in the region of 16mg. However, when used clinically to lower cholesterol, it is often taken in doses which are enormously larger – one to three *grams* – two hundred times the recommended daily allowance. Only niacin in its nicotinic acid form has been found useful to lower cholesterol; nicotinamide does not have the same effect.

For those people who suffer from very high blood cholesterol, doctors sometimes prescribe niacin combined with one or more other types of drug (perhaps something called a bile acid sequestrant, such as cholestyramine) and additional diet therapy. Under these conditions, it is not uncommon to find a huge reduction in cholesterol of 45 to 60 per cent!

You should remember, however, that your first line of attack against cholesterol should be to reduce your total and saturated fat and cholesterol intake, to control your weight, to increase your physical activity and to control any disease (such as diabetes or hypothyroidism) which may be elevating your cholesterol. The range of side-effects which have been associated with taking megadoses of niacin make it much less suitable than other, more natural, methods. Drug therapy (which is what taking large doses of niacin amounts to) should be used only when all these measures have failed, and under the supervision of your doctor.

Beans

Beans can be just as effective as oat bran in lowering cholesterol, because they contain useful amounts of the same soluble fibre; 100g of oat bran contain nearly 8g of soluble fibre. By using the following table, you can see how several different types of beans compare.[48]

Food	Grams of soluble fibre in 100g
Green beans, tinned	8.13
Navy beans, cooked	7.76
Pinto beans, cooked	7.52
Baked beans, tinned	6.3
Kidney beans, tinned	5.26

When researchers gave ten men suffering from high cholesterol a diet containing half a cup of tinned baked beans every day for three weeks, they found that cholesterol levels had dropped by an average of 13 per cent and triglycerides had sunk by 12 per cent.[49] And this was on an 'average' diet which included a considerable amount of dietary fat and cholesterol. When British researchers carried out similar experiments, they also found that beans could cut cholesterol levels by about one-third.[50] The researchers used plain, ordinary, tinned baked beans, and asked volunteers to eat one 500g tin per day. Within three days of starting, the subjects showed a 10 to 12 per cent drop in cholesterol! It seems, therefore, that eating some beans every day is a healthy, and easy, way to increase your cholesterol loss.

Rice bran

Recent research shows that rice bran (the stuff lost when converting brown rice to white rice) can be just as effective as oat bran in lowering cholesterol. But it may not work the same way. 'We just don't think rice bran works by the same mechanism as oat bran,' says Robin Saunders of the US Department of Agriculture. He believes the cholesterol-fighting agent in rice bran may be the oil it contains. Rice bran oil is high in b-sitosterol. It is thought that b-sitosterol and cholesterol compete for absorption in the intestines; therefore, an increased absorption of b-sitosterol means a decreased absorption of cholesterol. Rice bran oil has been widely used by Japanese cooks for 50 years and is starting to become available in the West.

Just a few years ago, it was thought that surgery was the only way to temporarily undo the damage that cholesterol could do to our circulation. But now we know that simply changing your lifestyle (reducing stress, lowering cholesterol levels) can effectively reverse heart disease. The evidence is there – let's act on it!

LifePoints Power Foods: Chronic Fatigue

Chronic Fatigue Syndrome (CFS), Myalgic Encephalomyelitis (ME), Postviral Syndrome (PVS), Chronic Monoycleosis-Like Syndrome or Chronic Epstein-Barr Virus Syndrome – whatever you call it, it's a debilitating disease which is still creating enormous controversy amongst orthodox medical practitioners. At the heart of CFS lies a severe disabling fatigue, lasting for at least six months, with a variety of other symptoms, including recurrent sore throats, headaches, muscle and joint pain, low fever, lymph-node swelling, intestinal discomfort and depression. The symptoms of CFS can last an average of 3½ to 4 years. Many people tend to get somewhat better after a year or so, but only 15 to 20 per cent of CFS patients seem to recover fully and 5 per cent remain homebound or bedridden.[51]

People with CFS are sometimes dismissed by doctors as hypochondriacs. While it is true that most sufferers do have an accompanying psychological disorder – usually depression – it is quite wrong to label the illness as 'psychosomatic' simply because of this. In America, the Centers for Disease Control now recognize CFS as a disease and are spending $1.5 million to study its frequency and impact.

Currently, there is no real laboratory test for CFS, although one may be on the horizon. Researchers in America have identified an abnormal level of certain white blood cells in people with CFS. These cells are known as CD8+ cytotoxic T-cells (T-cells help the immune system fight infection). Along with a high level of CD8+ cytotoxic T-cells, researchers have found a low level of CD8+ 'suppressor' cells.[52] A future laboratory test could conceivably be based on these findings. Normally, CFS is only diagnosed when other illnesses – such as anaemia, cancer, depression, diabetes and allergies – have been ruled out. A physical examination and routine laboratory tests often reveal nothing, and blood tests fail to show up any viral infection. Part of the difficulty with diagnosis is tied up with the vagueness of the very definition of 'fatigue' and the wide range of symptoms involved.

CFS seems particularly to target 'overachievers' in the 20 to 40 age group. That's why it has cruelly been called 'yuppie flu', because it so often affects successful people. This glib term fails to take into account the very real severity and length of the illness.

The cause of CFS is still basically unknown, but a number of theories have been suggested. One theory proposes that it may be caused by chronic infection with Epstein-Barr virus (EBV). Part of the herpes group of viruses, EBV can produce a lifelong latent infection. Almost all of us have become infected by EBV by the time we are adults, but with a healthy immune system it will not become troublesome.[53] However, CFS has not been consistently linked with Epstein-Barr (or any other virus) and the American Centers for Disease Control have now dropped the EBV label.

Another theory involves overgrowth of the common yeast *Candida albicans*. Candida is normally present in every person's body and can sometimes cause minor infections of the mucus membranes of the mouth or vagina (thrush). With a healthy immune system, candida causes few problems, because it is kept under control. However, with a weakened immune system, candida may flourish, creating symptoms similar to CFS. The idea that CFS might be connected to candida infection was first proposed in 1977 by C. Orian Truss, MD, a certified internist from Birmingham, Alabama.[54] Truss found that many of his chronically ill patients improved on a treatment regime which featured a sugar-free, yeast-free diet and nystatin, a safe anti-fungal medication taken by mouth.

Apart from a malfunctioning immune system, other factors in the proliferation of candida may include the use of antibiotics, which, while killing both 'good' and 'bad' bacteria in the body indiscriminately, allow candida to grow unchecked. Says Dr Belinda Dawes, a British doctor who has specialized in the treatment of CFS:

> I would now say that without doubt, candida infection plays a rôle in the ill health of all of the patients I see. Although their illness may not be directly related to the candida problem, eliminating the candida from their body and its related consequences has certainly been one of the factors in their recovery.[55]

However, the candida/CFS connection is by no means accepted by all doctors. At least one study has failed to show any benefit at all to CFS sufferers from taking anti-fungal drugs such as nystatin.[56]

Dr Peter Nixon, a cardiologist at London's Charing Cross Hospital, has attracted much controversy by stating his belief that CFS is simply a result of chronic exhaustion:

> We're always getting fashionable diseases – ten years ago it was total allergy syndrome. Then it was spasmophilia. After

that it was food allergy – have you noticed how that's fading away? Now it's ME. To my mind they're all basically the same – people have got into terrible fatigue and they can't get out. Nowadays, people simply aren't allowed to be tired. Yet nobody can do a high performance job, working 14 hours a day, for ever. We have to behave like winning people all the time – and our systems can't stand it.[57]

Some researchers even believe that the epidemic of Chronic Fatigue Syndrome may be related to the AIDS epidemic. Brain scans of some CFS patients show the same abnormalities as those seen in scans of patients with AIDS. More than 100 physicians and 3000 nurses have come down with CFS, and almost all of them have treated patients with AIDS (they are not HIV positive).[58]

Ultimately, the root cause of CFS may well involve a wide combination of factors – environmental toxins, food allergens, activated viruses, a higher than normal presence of *Candida albicans*, lack of good-quality sleep and far too much prolonged stress.

What can you do?

Because the root cause hasn't yet been pinpointed, conventional medical treatment is directed towards alleviating the most distressing symptoms. But most studies have generally had little success using drugs such as anti-inflammatories, antibiotics, tranquillizers or anti-herpes medicines.

- First, get a thorough medical check-up, in order to exclude treatable, physical or psychological problems that may be producing the symptoms. An underactive thyroid, problems with the temporomandibular joint (TMJ, the jaw joint), parasite and yeast infections, mitral valve prolapse (incomplete closing of a heart valve), sugar intolerance and low blood sugar, and various allergies and hypersensitivities to food and environmental substances can all produce symptoms similar to CFS.[59]
- Many CFS patients respond well to a diet of natural, unprocessed foods with lots of fibre and plant food and very little fat. Protein is kept to a minimum and around ten glasses of water are drunk every day.

- Dr Jesse Stoff, a consultant in viro-immunology and also a qualified homeopath, believes that patients with CFS should try to sleep from 9 p.m. to 3 a.m., because it is during this time that the liver regenerates its exhausted Kupffer cells, which are vital to the body's immunological function.[60] Stoff also recommends a wholefood diet together with extensive dietary supplementation, including zinc, selenium, magnesium, beta-carotene, vitamin C, calcium lactate and vitamin B complex.

- A detoxification diet to remove all obstacles to health – both internal and external toxins – is a vital step towards achieving optimum immunity. A good naturopath or homeopath will be able to individually prescribe the right detoxification programme for your own personal requirements.

- Certain herbal medicines may be useful in stimulating the immune system and thus overcoming fatigue. These should be used under the supervision of a qualified herbalist:

  1 Pokeweed (*Phytolacca decandra Americana*) can improve immunological response and act as an antiviral agent.

  2 Liquorice root (*Glycyrrhiza glabra*) is useful for its antiviral activity.

  3 *Radix astragalus* has long been known for its rôle in strengthening the body's resistance, particularly in wasting and exhausting diseases.

  4 *Lomatium dissectum* and *Ligusticum porteri* are both used in Native American and naturopathic medicine to treat viral infections. Although there is no specific research to indicate their value in viral-related infections, there is a great deal of empirical evidence to suggest their role in treating CFS.

  5 Shiitake mushroom (*Lentinus edodes*) has always been used in traditional Chinese medicine to help improve resistance to disease. It has been found to contain a complex which stimulates the immune system while remaining non-toxic.

LifePoints Power Foods: Common Cold

The common cold is the most widespread illness in Western countries. The average child gets about six colds a year, while adults get two or three colds annually.[61] What can we do to defeat this minor but most exasperating illness? Here are some diet strategies that are worth trying.

The foods you eat can be used both to prevent and to treat the dreaded sniffles, aches and chills of the common cold. A lucky 6 to 10 per cent of the population never get colds; and by changing your diet you could become one of them. A cold is a viral infection, caused by any one of an estimated 200 different cold viruses. Each virus produces its own slightly different set of symptoms, which may include headache, chills, catarrh, sore throat, swollen glands and general malaise. Although not normally serious, colds can sometimes lead on to respiratory disorders, pneumonia and meningitis. Some people still think that colds are brought about by cold weather, but a more logical explanation is that in winter we are in poorer health with a lower resistance to infection. During the colder months, we do less exercise, eat fewer fruits and vegetables and generally take less care of ourselves.

Getting rid of a cold

When your nose streams or you cough violently, it is for a reason. Your body is doing all it can to rid itself of the things making it feel so terrible in the first place. Most of the concoctions you can buy over the counter just suppress these symptoms and do not actually help treat your cold. A much more successful approach is to assist your body in its battle.

- Drink plenty of clear, unsweetened liquids during a cold. Do not drink honey and lemon, orange juice or other naturally sweet beverages. Although it is popularly supposed that honey will soothe your throat and fruit juice will give you vitamin C, in fact honey, citrus fruits and any other form of sugar or sweet food can diminish the functioning of your immune system and so make it more difficult for your body to fight the virus.
- There is evidence that both the duration and severity of the common cold can be reduced by vitamin C intake.[62] [63] Linus Pauling, pioneer of orthomolecular medicine, suggests you should take two 1000 mg (1g) tablets of vitamin C at the first sign of a cold (scratchy throat, mucus in the nose, etc.) and that this dose should be repeated every hour for several

hours. If the symptoms persist, Pauling suggests a total intake of 10–20g of vitamin C per day to cure it. Foods especially rich in vitamin C include blackcurrants, citrus fruits, strawberries, cauliflower, cabbage and Brussels sprouts.

- Several scientific studies have shown that zinc can be useful in reducing the duration of a cold. In one study, a group of volunteers, all suffering from colds, were given a lozenge to suck every two hours while they were awake. Some of the lozenges contained 23mg of zinc gluconate, others contained none (a placebo). After seven days, it was found that 86 per cent of the group sucking the zinc lozenges had been cured, while only 46 per cent of those sucking the placebos were without cold symptoms. The researchers concluded that the zinc lozenges shortened the average duration of colds by about seven days.[64] Side-effects were usually minor and consisted mainly of objectionable taste and mouth irritation, but this high dose of zinc should not be taken for more than a few days. Foods naturally rich in zinc include pumpkin and sunflower seeds, nuts, wholemeal bread, mushrooms, soybeans and brewers' yeast. Here is a quick recipe that will help you get a strong dose of zinc – deliciously!

Roasted Pumpkin Seeds

Heat a large frying pan over a medium flame. Measure 115g (4 oz) of raw, shelled pumpkin seeds and pour into the pan. Keep the pan over the heat, shaking or stirring constantly while the seeds roast and pop. After 4–5 minutes, pour one tablespoon of shoyu or tamari (soy sauce) over the seeds. Stir quickly, remove from the heat and turn into a serving bowl. Allow to cool before eating.

- A fever is one of your body's weapons, an attempt to heat infection out of your system; when allowed to run its course a fever is usually successful. Do not try to suppress a fever unless your temperature rises above 104 °F (40 °C). And try this favoured home remedy: boil a handful of dried yarrow herb in 1 l (2 pints) of water, keeping the pan covered and simmering for 30 minutes. Serve in half-cupfuls every 30 minutes to promote sweating. Keep well wrapped up and warm during this time.

- Extra rest and sleep are *essential* to shake off a cold virus.
- Short-term fasting can help to boost your immune system when it is under attack (for example, when you've got a cold coming on). Studies show that fasting for up to 36 hours can increase the number of active phagocytes (which form the first line of defence against infection) in your body by up to 50 per cent.[65] But don't go beyond this time limit when you're ill, otherwise your immune system may not be able to cope.
- Eat plenty of garlic. Garlic has a long history of use in fighting infection and improving resistance to disease. You may enjoy the health-giving effects of garlic without the odour (if you find it objectionable) by preparing the following recipe:

Garlic Soup

Coarsely chop 12 to 15 cloves of garlic, including their skins, and place in a saucepan with one medium potato, cubed, and 1 l (2 pints) boiling water. Cover and simmer gently for 40 minutes. Add freshly grated ginger if desired. Drink one cupful every two hours if you feel the early symptoms of a cold.

- Eat between two and five umeboshi plums each day. These are a form of pickled plum originating in China and Japan which have a long and remarkable history of fighting infection. Buy them from Japanese supermarkets or your local health food shop. Available in paste or concentrate form as well.

LIFEPOINTS POWER FOODS: CONSTIPATION

Are you constipated at the moment? Four people out of every ten in the United Kingdom will answer 'Yes' to that question. In 20 per cent of the population, constipation is so severe that laxatives are used regularly. It is a startling fact that 77 per cent of the population only excrete between five and seven stools per week. That's over three-quarters of the total population! On top of that, a further 8 per cent of people only pass three or four stools a week. That makes 85 per cent of us with sluggish bowel movements.[66] Clearly, it's a national epidemic!

Chronic constipation occurs when you retain your stools in the colon and rectum so that the water they naturally contain is reabsorbed by the body. The stools then harden even more, making defecation more difficult. Eventually, your bowel loses its muscle tone and constipation becomes a way of life. Conventional medicine treats the symptom of constipation and brings about short-term purgative relief through the use of laxatives. However, the cause of constipation is what really needs treating in order to bring about a lasting solution to the problem. Constipation can be a symptom of a great many diseases; but for most of us the underlying cause is in our diets.

Good and bad foods

- Cut back on foods which slow down the passage of food through the body. These include fatty food such as meat, cheese and other animal produce, refined foods such as sugar and white flour, and most processed foods.
- Increase those foods which are good for your digestion and can speed up the process. You'll be pleased to know that as you do this you'll also be cutting back on your risk of developing cancer, heart disease and other killers of our Western civilization. Fruits, vegetables, pulses and whole grains are all fibre-rich foods. Start these simple changes to your diet now, and you will find an effective, long-term and natural cure for constipation.
- Beetroot juice – either bottled or freshly juiced – is a very useful short-term natural stool softener and laxative.

Much heaving and straining could be prevented if we only ate a diet that was higher in natural forms of fibre! Oat bran, baked beans, pumpkin seeds, wheat fibre, bran and all the bran products, these are all excellent sources of dietary fibre. Porridge for breakfast, lots of wholewheat products and one main meal consisting of a raw salad will significantly boost your fibre intake. The evidence shows that it will also prevent problems like haemorrhoids and diverticular diseases.

A salad with get up and go!

There is nothing more boring on the face of the earth than a traditional salad consisting of a few leaves of lettuce well past their sell-by date and accompanied by squishy but tasteless tomatoes. Yuk! This is how to make a proper salad.

Salad

Ingredients: tin of kidney beans, carrots, beetroot, cabbage, watercress, broccoli, potatoes, tofu, sunflower seeds, almonds, pumpkin seeds; plus any seasonal vegetables, including winter roots. Perm any six from ten! There's no need for lettuce, but make it a cos if you want it: it's got some flavour and it won't go limp.

Get a really large bowl. Cube the potatoes and lightly steam them and the broccoli; roast the pumpkin seeds; cube the tofu; grate the raw carrot and beetroot (don't slice); thin-shred the cabbage; fine-chop the watercress; wash and roughly chop the lettuce; don't forget the sunflower seeds and almonds. All this is quick to do, but get a food processor if you want to speed it up even more.

Prepare your favourite dressing. Two suggestions: olive oil, cider vinegar and French mustard (real French mustard please, no appalling English substitutes); or, for the most unusual dressing you've ever tasted – try this and you'll never try anything else! – buy some powdered black salt from your local Indian deli. Add two teaspoonsful to oil and cider vinegar, shake thoroughly until dissolved.

Place the lettuce in the bottom and round the side of the bowl, if you're using lettuce. Mix the other ingredients together and put them on top. Pour on the dressing.

One serving of a salad like this will give you a third of your total daily requirement of protein, almost twice your vitamin A requirement, all your vitamin C, and half your iron and fibre. It's so good you'll want to eat it every day! Tofu and, even nicer, marinated tofu are both available from health food shops.

Finally, don't get hooked on laxatives. If you're already taking them, try to get off. Although a natural laxative can be useful for a few days' short-term usage – for example, if you've been abroad on a different diet, and your bowels are suffering from culture shock – all laxatives have some kind of side-effects and they all subvert the natural processes of your body. Eventually, your bowels become dependent on them for a jump-start every day.

LifePoints Power Foods: Diabetes

Diabetes is a disease of the Western world, brought about by both genetic and environmental factors. In the UK alone nearly 1 million men, women and children are diabetic; worldwide an estimated 30 million people are known to suffer from diabetes. Diabetes mellitus is 'a disorder in which the body is unable to control the amount of sugar in the blood, because the mechanism which converts sugar to energy is no longer functioning properly'.[67]

Normally, the food you eat is gradually broken down and converted to glucose (blood sugar), the source of energy for all your body's functions. The conversion of glucose into energy requires insulin, a hormone produced in the pancreas. Insulin is released into your system in order to control the level of glucose in your blood, especially to prevent your blood sugar level from climbing too high. However, in diabetics there is either a shortage of insulin or the available insulin does not function as it should. The result is that glucose is not converted into energy, but builds up in the blood and eventually spills over into your urine. This is often one of the first signs of diabetes.

Though there is an abundance of glucose in your blood, the body is still deprived of the energy it needs (because the glucose has not been converted to energy) and so the liver begins to produce yet more glucose to meet demands. Shortly, your body's stores of fat and protein begin to break down in another attempt to supply more glucose. The resulting weight loss is often a further sign of diabetes. Thus begins a chain of events within your body that can eventually cause severe health problems, even death. In the UK alone, approximately 20,000 people die prematurely each year from diabetes-related problems.[68]

Diabetes sufferers are of two types. Those who are insulin dependent produce little or no insulin in their body and require injections of insulin to survive. This type of diabetes is sometimes called Type 1 or 'juvenile-onset' diabetes. Those who are non-insulin dependent produce some insulin in their body but it is not sufficient or does not function to maintain good health. This is sometimes called Type 2 or 'maturity-onset' diabetes.

Diabetes is a serious disorder and unfortunately its incidence is increasing – in Britain an estimated 60,000 new cases are diagnosed each year.[69] Further, the number of children diagnosed as diabetic has doubled in the past 20 years and this appears to be a worldwide trend. In short, this problem is getting worse. But there are simple, effective steps which you can take to prevent the onset of diabetes or minimize its erosion of your health if you already have it.

Prevent or cure?

According to a report submitted by Diabetes Epidemiology Research International (DERI) to the *British Medical Journal*,[70] between 60 and 95 per cent of cases of insulin-dependent diabetes can be prevented. The DERI group of scientists believe that environmental factors are largely responsible for the increase in diabetes, claiming that genetic factors could not account for such great increases over such a very short period of time. Of the possible environmental causes, diet is perhaps the most significant and certainly one over which we have control.

Further, it seems that the same dietary measures used in the prevention of diabetes can be used with great success in treatment. There have been several clues pointing to this possibility. For instance, Nauru, a remote island in the Pacific, had never had any cases of diabetes until it suddenly became rich and began to import American-style fast food. Now, more than 40 per cent of its population over the age of 20 have diabetes! Similarly, diabetes is noticeably rare in parts of Africa and China where the traditional diet is intact and free from Western influence. So what are the dietary influences which can prevent or treat diabetes?

- The American Diabetes Association suggests that diabetics eat a diet in which carbohydrates make up about 60 per cent of total calorie intake, these carbohydrates to be mostly unrefined, complex and high in fibre.[71] Fat intake should total less than 30 per cent of calories consumed, with an emphasis on reducing saturated fats and cholesterol, replacing them with monounsaturated fats such as olive oil. Protein intake should be moderate.
- Avoid eating meat. Diabetes is more common among meat-eating people than non-meat-eaters. Meat-eating increases consumption of saturated fats, which may affect insulin sensitivity. Also, the N-nitroso compounds in meat may actually be a trigger to the development of diabetes.

In a 21-year study of 25,698 adult Seventh Day Adventists, it was found that they were less than half (45 per cent) as likely to suffer diabetes as an underlying cause of death than the rest of the population.[72] Seventh Day Adventists avoid consuming meat, fish, eggs, coffee, alcohol and tobacco. When other factors were taken into account, the study found that 'a vegetarian diet reduces the risk of developing diabetes'.[73] That means that if you are vegetarian you are less likely to develop diabetes in the first place.

- Replace meat with protein foods such as whole grains, nuts, seeds, tofu, pulses, Quorn and soya products. In addition to meeting your protein needs, these foods contain valuable vitamins, minerals and fibre – something meat hasn't got!

- A high-fat diet is already implicated in other serious diseases such as stroke and heart disease. But too much fat in the diet also contributes to obesity; many diabetics are obese, which further complicates their disorder. Start by replacing saturated fats such as butter with cold-pressed vegetable oils and cut down on dairy products generally. These are obvious sources of fat, but many packaged, frozen or highly processed foods contain hidden fats which quickly and quietly boost your calorie count. So eat fresh produce wherever possible, and, when cooking, avoid frying or roasting; steam, bake or boil instead.

- A high-fibre diet can lower the amount of insulin you need to inject (if you are insulin dependent) and can eliminate the need for insulin in some Type 2 diabetics. Select foods high in fibre, especially soluble fibre, such as whole grains, beans, oats, bran and vegetables.

- Coffee can raise the concentration of sugar in the blood. As this is the major symptom of diabetes, coffee consumption may have serious implications for diabetics and potential diabetics alike. If you drink large amounts of coffee while pregnant, your children become more susceptible to diabetes.[74]

- Diabetics are commonly lacking in vitamin B6, which is vital for insulin production. So give preference to foods in your diet which are rich in vitamin B6 – oat bran and oat germ, avocados, bananas, brewers' yeast, yeast extract, brown rice, parsley, spinach and other green leafy vegetables, molasses and whole grains.

- Vitamin C is needed to metabolize insulin and glucose; a deficiency can lead to cell degeneration in the pancreas, where insulin is produced. Eat plenty of citrus fruits, alfalfa sprouts and vegetables such as potato, green pepper and broccoli. As the body cannot store vitamin C, there is no danger of toxicity from supplementation should you wish to take a high-dose vitamin C tablet every day.

- Diabetics often have a deficiency in the trace mineral chromium and can benefit from supplementation, with elderly and non-insulin-dependent diabetics responding particularly well. Chromium acts with insulin to transport glucose through cell walls. Highly processed foods always have reduced levels of chromium and years of eating such foods can invite the onset of Type 2, maturity-onset, diabetes. A diet rich in chromium may prevent this. Eat plenty of wheat germ, brewers' yeast, whole grains and corn oil.

- Zinc plays a crucial role in the synthesis and storage of insulin in the pancreas. It is a mineral that many of us, not just diabetics, are continually short of. Eat mushrooms, sunflower and pumpkin seeds, brewers' yeast and soybeans to boost your zinc intake.

- Foods rich in magnesium may help to prevent retinopathy, a deterioration of the retina which is a real threat to diabetics. Foods rich in magnesium include nuts, whole grains, dark green vegetables and molasses.

LIFEPOINTS POWER FOODS: ECZEMA AND PSORIASIS

As a sufferer you will know the red, scaly, often painful skin which typifies psoriasis and eczema. Both are chronic, non-contagious skin disorders which affect people of all ages. The joints, scalp, back, chest, bottom, hands and legs, and in acute cases virtually the whole body, can be affected. Both conditions can be brought on by allergy, stress, anxiety, viruses, flu, overtiredness or injury – especially if you have a history of either disorder in the family. Rather than accept your problem as inevitable, however, you can make changes in your diet which will minimize or solve your skin problem.

- Adopt a low-sugar or even a sugar-free diet to prevent an overgrowth of the *Candida albicans* yeast in your gut. This yeast is normally present in a healthy person but, when present to excess, can cause disease or reduced immunity. Psoriasis is particularly responsive to a reduction in your sugar intake and a few days or weeks on a sugar-free diet (sometimes called an anti-fungal diet) may improve your condition.[75] Remember, sugar includes honey, molasses, concentrated fruit juices and syrups.

- Adopt a dairy- and gluten-free diet for two to three weeks to determine whether your skin problem is aggravated by these food groups.

- In some people, a deficiency in the B-complex of vitamins can hinder the proper metabolism of fats and proteins, and problems such as psoriasis and eczema can result. To correct deficiency, you may take a B-complex supplement daily. Simply ensure that your supplement includes the whole range of B vitamins as they work best when taken as a group. The B vitamins are essential to the health of skin, mucus membranes and nerves. In fact, as stress is so often a trigger for eczema and psoriasis, a sufficiency of the B-complex may help prevent an attack by reducing the initial effects of stress on your body.

  Foods especially rich in the B-complex are yeasts, such as brewers' or nutritional yeast, and whole grains. Pulses and seeds are also useful sources. Ensure that you have a serving of each of these foods in your diet each day.

- Gamma-linolenic acid is a substance which we produce in our bodies. Some people, however, do not produce enough and are more likely to suffer from eczema as a result. A bowl of porridge each day is a good source of gamma-linolenic acid,[76] as is a supplement in the form of evening primrose oil.[77] This supplement is available both over the counter from health food shops and on prescription through the NHS.

- Omega-3 fatty acids reduce the itching and scaling of eczema and psoriasis in many people.[78] Sources of omega-3 fatty acids include flaxseed or soya oils, which you may take as supplements.

- Selenium and vitamin E are both antioxidants and work together to preserve and promote healthy metabolic processes. Of particular importance to sufferers of eczema and psoriasis, this combination can delay the oxidation of essential fatty acids which are so crucial to healthy skin. Selenium is a mineral found in whole grains, especially the bran and germ, and vegetables such as onions, celery, cabbage and broccoli. Vitamin E is abundant in cold-pressed vegetable oils, in soybeans and in all raw nuts and seeds.

- A poorly functioning digestive system results in the proliferation of various toxins within the gut. Several of these toxins can contribute to the development of psoriasis and eczema.[79] There are several dietary steps you may take to improve digestion and therefore prevent or minimize your skin problem.

- Take a supplement of *Lactobacillus acidophilus*, a friendly bacterium which will colonize your gut and help to correct many digestive disorders.

- Increase your intake of dietary fibre. Start by altering your diet to include an abundance of fresh fruit and vegetables as well as two or three servings daily of whole, unprocessed grains.

- Boost your intake of folic acid as some psoriasis sufferers have been shown to have low blood levels of folic acid.[80] Folic acid is found in green leafy vegetables and brewers' yeast.

- Zinc is essential for the production of hydrochloric acid in your stomach, a shortage of which produces digestive problems which can lead to eczema or psoriasis. Zinc is found in whole grains, pumpkin seeds and brewers' yeast.

- Vitamin A is necessary for the health of all body tissue, especially the skin and mucus membranes. Skin problems such as eczema and psoriasis can be one sign of deficiency and may respond well to increased intakes of vitamin A or carotene, the vegetable substance which your body converts to vitamin A. To boost your intake of vitamin A, eat plenty of carotene-rich foods, including dark green leafy vegetables, such as spinach, and vegetables of a dark orange colour such as carrots and pumpkin.

- Some people's eczema or psoriasis is an allergic response. If you suspect this might be true for you, try amending your diet in these ways:
  1 Eat only fresh, organic produce to avoid chemical residues and unnecessary additives.
  2 Eliminate the foods which most commonly cause an allergic response. These include dairy products, eggs,

fish, peanuts and soybeans.[81] Other foods, such as chicken, citrus, tomato and corn, may also cause an allergic response.

3 Adopt a vegetarian or vegan diet for six to eight weeks. Some people have experienced an improvement in their health as a result of this type of diet.[82]

- Moderately high alcohol consumption can aggravate psoriasis. A Finnish study[83] concluded that men who consumed 5 or more units of alcohol per day were likely to suffer a worsening of their condition. Try keeping your alcohol intake to the recommended 21 units per week for men, 14 units per week for women.

LIFEPOINTS POWER FOODS: FALLING HAIR

Male pattern baldness (MPB) is hereditary; and there's not much you can do about it, other than wear a toupee or have an expensive hair transplant. If a naked pate is your fate, accept it cheerfully. The human race has gradually lost its total body covering of hair since its furry primate days, and your own hairlessness is simply proof of your evolved nature – in a few millennia or so, everyone else will have caught up with you!

Women, of course, don't suffer from MPB, although it is quite common for pregnancy to produce temporary hair loss. Other possible causes of hair loss may include hormone deficiency, anaemia, illness, use of steroids, antibiotics, ringworm and, increasingly in today's world, stress.

Conventionally, there is little that orthodox medicine can do, other than investigate possible underlying causes such as skin conditions, scalp disorders and alopecia, and then refer you to a trichologist. So here are some natural alternatives to consider:

Minerals

There are certain minerals that are essential to hair growth. Zinc, in particular, has long been recognized as a means of promoting healthy hair and, more generally, zinc is essential for bodily healing. Smoking will definitely lower your zinc level – so stub it out. Keep your zinc levels high by eating fresh, leafy green vegetables like spinach, and eat lots of wholegrain products.

The trace mineral copper, too, is vital for healthy hair and skin. It prevents defects in hair colour and structure. Good sources of copper, as of zinc, are wholegrain cereals, especially quinoa. Eggs, cherries, nuts and beans are also copper sources.

Drugs

It's a little-known fact that many of the prescription and over-the-counter drugs used can and do cause temporary hair loss as one of their adverse effects. While individual reactions may vary from one person to another, this side-effect can occur with all the following drugs: cholesterol-lowering drugs, arthritis medications, beta-blocker blood pressure drugs, anti-ulcer drugs, oral contraceptives, blood thinners, epileptic medications, male hormones (anabolic steroids) and vitamin A-derived drugs. If you suspect your hair loss is linked to the medication you're taking, ask your doctor if another drug without this side-effect can be used instead.

Herbal remedies

Many of the foods traditionally used to combat falling hair are rubbed on, not eaten. An old recipe for a hair stimulant passed down amongst gypsies has it that 30g of rosemary should be boiled in a pint of water for five minutes and then rubbed into the scalp every night. And it's true that one rarely sees a bald gypsy.

A traditional French remedy for baldness involves massaging the scalp with freshly pressed nettle juice every night. To extract the juice, either use a modern juicing machine or pound the nettles in a mortar, then place them in a fine cloth and press well.

Another French folk remedy directs you to rub the scalp gently with olive oil, then go to bed with your head wrapped in a towel. Next morning, shampoo with tepid water and very simple soap. Repeat for ten consecutive days every month – preferably while the moon is waxing. Two beaten eggs can be substituted for the olive oil.

Food

A good, well-balanced diet, consisting of good protein sources like beans, pulses, grains and nuts, together with lots of fresh vegetables, will keep your hair healthy. Falling hair may be a sign of vitamin A deficiency or, paradoxically, of vitamin A overdose. The B group of vitamins, found in yeast products and wholegrain cereals, are also essential for good hair condition.

The Chinese eat one sheet of nori every day – a dried seaweed available in health food shops – in order to preserve the shiny black colour of their hair well into old age.

To make a superb hair tonic take a handful of rosemary and two cups of cider vinegar, and place in a covered pan over a low heat for one hour. Cool and strain. Shampoo your hair normally, rinse, then pour half a cup of the rosemary mixture over your scalp and leave for three minutes before rinsing it out.

LIFEPOINTS POWER FOODS: GALLSTONES

If you eat a diet low in saturated fats and refined sugar and high in fibre, your chances of developing gallstones are small. If, however, you eat a typical Western diet, that is lots of fat and refined foods, then you may be one of the 17 per cent of the population to discover 'gallstone hell'. And hell it is – the pain can be intense. It's like being kicked in the guts by a horse – all the time, as one sufferer has described it. As the Western diet has changed, so has the incidence of gallstones, quadrupling since 1940 in many areas. Orientals and rural Africans, who traditionally consume a low-fat, high-fibre diet, suffer from them very rarely. In addition, only humans and domesticated animals have gallstones; wild animals do not. This also strongly suggests that the problem is connected to our modern Western diets.

Gallstones are more common amongst women than men – 25 per cent of all women and 10 per cent of all men will develop gallstones before they are 60 years old. The overweight and diabetic are also more at risk. Gallstones form when the substances found in bile, such as cholesterol and calcium, begin to precipitate, forming stones which cause pain, nausea and vomiting. They can also lead to infection, resulting in inflammation of the gall bladder, colic, peritonitis, gangrene of the gall bladder and jaundice.

Protect against them

If you are obese you are four times more likely to suffer from stones. One more good reason to shed those kilograms – right? Well yes, but be careful how you diet. Rapid weight loss can actually *increase* your risk of suffering from gallstones (another good reason to follow the gradual weight-loss regime of *LifePoints Diet*). Obese people who lose a lot of weight on very low-calorie diets are quite likely to form stones. Once the weight has been lost, however, and relatively normal eating patterns are restored, the stones may dissolve of their own accord. It is best to have your doctor supervise this.

Taking oestrogen or oral contraceptives can increase the amount of cholesterol in your bile fluid and thus the chances of having gallstones. At least three studies have found an increased risk of gall bladder disease among women who use oral contraceptives.

If you are a meat-eater, you are doubling your chances of developing gallstones, according to one study carried out in Oxford.[84] Two groups of women were compared to see if their diets could have any influence on the occurrence of gallstones. The 632 women in the first group were selected at random and ate meat. The second group consisted of 130 women who did not eat meat and had a diet naturally higher in fibre. All the women were then given a thorough inspection, using ultrasound detection techniques, looking specifically for gallstones. The experimenters found that the meat-eaters were two and a half times more likely to develop gallstones than the non-meat-eaters. The scientists concluded that the low-fat, high-fibre diet of the non-meat-eating women gave them protection.

And survive in spite of them!

Once you've got gallstones, they're not easy to get rid of by dietary means alone. Conventional medicine can offer you a range of choices. Surgical removal of the stones or of the gallbladder itself is quite common, and people who have their gallbladder removed usually don't seem to suffer any adverse consequences. Another possible therapy is the use of chemical solvents to dissolve some kinds of stones. Finally, sound waves called extracorporeal shock wave lithotripsy, or ESWL, can crush the stones into smaller bits which can then be excreted.

Fatty foods are known to stimulate gallbladder contractions, which can cause a painful gallstone attack, yet another reason to eat a low-RiskPoints diet. Also, consuming smaller, more frequent meals may help limit gallbladder contractions and gallstone attacks.

Recently, there has been scientific speculation that a diet high in soluble fibre might increase the solubility of cholesterol in the bile and so prevent, perhaps even reverse, the formation of gallstones. Good sources of soluble fibre include oat bran, pectin, and beans. See 'LifePoints Power Foods: Cholesterol' (page 134) for more details.

LifePoints Power Foods: High Blood Pressure

Hypertension is the medical name for high blood pressure. Orthodox medicine has made impressive progress in the detection and treatment of hypertension, and this has resulted in a decline in mortality from strokes, for example, over the last three decades. But there's no room for complacency. Raised blood pressure is one of the key risk factors in the development of heart disease and cerebrovascular disease. The United Kingdom government estimates that over 240,000 people die every year as a result of a hypertension-related disease. Put another way, 33 per cent – one-third – of all deaths that occur in people aged less than 65 are attributable to hypertensive causes.

Blood pressure is measured by the height in millimetres of a column of mercury that can be raised inside a vacuum. The more pressure there is, the higher the column will rise. Since blood pressure varies with every heartbeat, two measures are taken – one measures the pressure of the beat itself (called systolic blood pressure) and the other measures the pressure in between beats, when the heart is resting (this is called diastolic blood pressure and is the 'background' level). These two figures are written with the systolic figure first, followed by the diastolic figure: 120/80.

When we're born, our systolic blood pressure is about 40, then it doubles to about 80 within the first month. Thereafter, the increase is slower, but inexorable, for the rest of our lives. Many people do not realize they suffer from hypertension. There may be no symptoms, and it may only be discovered during a visit to the doctor's surgery for another complaint. In its later stages symptoms may include headache, dizziness, fatigue and insomnia.

A pressure of 150/90 would be considered high in a young person, and 160/95 would be abnormally high. In older people, systolic pressure could be 140 at age 60, and 160 at age 80 years.

Symptoms of high blood pressure (hypertension) include dizziness, headaches, irritability and fatigue. There is also a real danger, even if you only suffer from a mild form, that it may develop into life-threatening illnesses and events such as heart attack, stroke and kidney disease. Treatment – whether through drugs or otherwise – ideally aims to reduce diastolic pressure to round about 80–85 mmHg.

What you can do

A diagnosis of high blood pressure is not a death sentence. There is a lot you can do to bring it down – providing you are willing to try seriously. Much research now clearly shows that many 'hypertensives' can lower their blood pressure by amending their lifestyle and dietary habits.

- Get to understand your own blood pressure. A device which measures blood pressure is called a 'sphygmomanometer', and consists of an inflatable cuff that is wrapped around the arm, connected via a tube to the measuring device. Simple sphygmomanometers are quite cheap, and it could be worth buying one and tracking your blood pressure as it rises and falls over a period of time. Blood pressure fluctuates considerably even in normal individuals – the reading taken at the doctor's surgery won't be the same as the one when you're at home later in the day. Physical activity, excitement, fear or emotional stress can all send it shooting up. The term 'hypertension' indicates that blood pressure exceeds the upper limits most of the time, not just for short periods. When you understand how your blood pressure changes, you're on the way to controlling it.

- One recent study has found that as many as 20 per cent of patients treated for hypertension could be receiving unnecessary medication, simply because their blood pressure rises in the presence of a doctor. They coined the term 'white coat hypertension' for this phenomenon.[85] With your own sphygmomanometer, you'll be able to rule this out in your case.

- Drugs should not be a first-resort measure for those who suffer from high blood pressure. It is now increasingly widely accepted that doctors should have patients with high blood pressure follow a strict diet, lose weight if necessary and exercise more to see if it improves their condition before prescribing drugs. Dr Rose Stamler, a Chicago epidemiologist, has reported that 40 per cent of patients manage to control their high blood pressure with moderate exercise and dietary modifications alone.[86]

- Normalize your weight. Most hypertensives are overweight, yet a 20 lb reduction in weight can result in a blood pressure reduction of 20 mmHg and 10 mmHg diastolic.[87]

- Reduce or avoid alcohol consumption. Most long-term studies have shown that blood pressure can be reduced significantly by cutting out or cutting down on the amount of alcohol consumed. For example, one study shows that among women taking more than two alcoholic drinks per day, one-third of all cases of hypertension are caused by alcohol consumption. This suggests that hypertension in these women may be treatable by restriction of alcohol intake.[88]

- Stop smoking. Nicotine stimulates the heart and at the same time constricts the blood vessels – making it difficult for your blood pressure not to rise! If you are a man with high blood pressure and you smoke, you are three and a half times more likely to develop cardiovascular disease than if you were a healthy non-smoker.

- Learn to relax and to exercise. Both of these activities help you to feel more in control of your body and your life.

- Consider a drastic change at work. People in demanding jobs with little freedom to make decisions have three times the risk of developing high blood pressure compared to others who have either a less demanding job or more decision-making latitude.[89]

- Eat from the first four LifePoints foods groups only. A group of long-term hypertensives on medication ate like this for one year. In almost all cases their medication was withdrawn or greatly reduced and they all claimed to feel better. More importantly, they enjoyed a decrease in blood pressure and many additional symptoms disappeared. Their diet was free of all animal products, i.e. meat, fish, eggs and dairy products.[90]

- Eat a high-fibre diet. Fibre guards against the hypertensive effects of fatty foods. In a three-day test, people with a high fibre intake had a lower mean blood pressure than those eating less fibre. When fibre was reduced in their diet, their blood pressure rose. High-fibre foods include whole grains, pulses, fruit and fresh vegetables.[91]

- Thirty couples in an area of East Finland with a very high level of coronary heart disease changed their normal high-fat and low-polyunsaturate diet to one lower in total and saturated fats – more similar to a low-RiskPoints diet. After only six weeks, they enjoyed a significant drop in blood pressure. Consumption of olive oil, a monounsaturated fat, is more strongly correlated to lower blood pressure than that of polyunsaturated oils.[92]

- Adjust your sodium and potassium intake. Both of these minerals are salts (sodium is table salt), which regulate the balance of fluid in your body. An excess of sodium increases the volume of blood, which puts more strain on the circulatory system, causing high blood pressure. Thus sodium has been blamed for many cases of hypertension. However, it is now shown that potassium can protect from hypertension because it balances the effects of sodium.[93] You can reduce your intake of sodium and increase your intake of potassium by limiting the amount of processed foods you eat – these are high in sodium and low in potassium. Instead, eat potassium-rich foods such as banana, broccoli, Brussels sprouts, dates, prunes and raisins. Jacket potatoes and cantaloupes are also good sources.

- Increase your intake of magnesium. The mineral is lost when you take diuretics – often prescribed for hypertensives. Yet 50 per cent of magnesium-deficient patients have high blood pressure, usually normalizing when this deficiency is rectified. Foods rich in magnesium include green vegetables, nuts, whole grains and yeast extracts.[94]

- Boost your calcium intake. It has been found that people with high blood pressure often have low levels of calcium.[95] In one study, researchers demonstrated a 23 per cent decrease in hypertension risk among women receiving 800mg per day of calcium, compared with women consuming just 400mg per day (the recommended daily allowance for adults is 800mg per day, 1200mg for pregnant or lactating women).[96] Foods rich in calcium include dairy products, tofu, spinach, figs, molasses, seaweeds, nuts and seeds, watercress and parsley.

LIFEPOINTS POWER FOODS: HYPERACTIVE CHILDREN

Hyperactivity – sometimes called Attention-Deficit Hyperactivity

Disorder (AHDH) – is an increasingly widespread problem among children. It arouses great medical controversy, because it is so difficult to give the condition a specific definition – one person's 'emotional disturbance' is another 'spoiled child'. One fact's for sure – if your child exhibits more than half of the following behaviour patterns there is cause for concern:

- Easy distraction
- Short attention span
- Difficulty following instructions
- Constant fidgeting or squirming
- Never completing an activity
- Excessive chattering and shouting out in class
- Constantly interrupting, not listening
- Wild and dangerous play
- Inability to play alone or quietly
- Disrupting others
- Excessive impatience.

Hyperactivity is a uniquely individual condition, and no single cause is likely to apply to all children affected. Broadly, possible causes fall into four major groupings:

- Genetic: an inherited tendency to hyperactivity. It is also speculated that excess alcohol consumption during pregnancy may predispose the child to later hyperactive behaviour.
- Medical: head injury, mental illness, sight and hearing problems, meningitis and hypoglycaemia can all result in hyperactive behaviour.
- Environmental: social upheaval, family breakdown and disturbed homelife, and lead poisoning may all be factors.
- School-related: hyperactivity which is brought on by academic failure, stress, lack of rapport with teachers or antagonism within the class situation.

Conventional medicine has developed a 'pill for every ill' attitude which is only recently being challenged by a younger and more open-minded generation of doctors. It is not surprising to learn, therefore, that several drugs exist which are claimed to be effective in the treatment of hyperactive children. In the United States, the most popular drug is methylphenidate, and it is estimated that over 750,000 children are currently receiving treatment.[97] Paradoxically, methylphenidate is actually a stimulant, which seems to have the incidental effect of slowing down hyperactive children. According to an article in the *Journal of the American Medical Association*, well over a million children are now estimated to receive stimulant drugs to 'treat' hyperactivity and classroom inattentiveness.[98] It is sadly ironic that, as the war against illegal stimulant drugs becomes ever more intense, doctors are busier than ever before prescribing legal stimulant drugs to young children and teenagers.

Increasingly, however, there is evidence to show that individual cases of hyperactivity are related to factors which are controllable without resorting to drugs.

Allergic reactions

Try these suggestions:

- In the home. Watch your child and keep a note of the severity of the symptoms from day to day. Does he or she appear more symptom-free when away from home? Does he or she seem more hyperactive, say, in cold weather when increasingly housebound? If so, then your child could be allergic to something in your home. Possibilities include dust, feathers, pets, mould spores, odours, chemicals; the list is endless. If you have grounds for suspicion, your doctor will be able to recommend a consultation with an allergy specialist, and skin tests can determine the answer.

- Outside. Check the pollen calendar. If a higher count relates to hyper-behaviour, a connection is worth considering. At school, is your child's behaviour worse by lunchtime or when he or she returns home after class? There are a myriad possibilities, ranging from allergy to an element in school lunches, through certain classrooms (like the gym, metal/woodwork room, art/cookery class) to heating/cleaning materials. They all have to be investigated, with the help of a friendly teacher.

- Food. This is the big one! A number of studies have been conducted which point the finger at a causal relationship between diet and hyperactivity. For example, a 1985 study at Great Ormond Street Hospital suggested that food additives such as tartrazine could seriously affect children's behaviour.[99] Seventy-six children who had been clinically diagnosed as hyperactive were treated with a simple, bland diet which contained none of the usual substances associated with hyperactivity. After treatment, 62 of the children had noticeably improved, and in 21 of them the symptoms of hyperactivity had entirely disappeared. The researchers found that artificial food colourings and food preservatives were the ingredients most likely to provoke bouts of hyperactivity. Some parents have also noticed that consumption of brightly coloured sweets and fizzy drinks transforms the behaviour of their kids. One mother compared her son to the 'Incredible Hulk' after he ate foods containing additives. Tartrazine is already banned in some countries. Other studies have caused suspicion to be cast on sugar, caffeine and cow's milk.

Criminologists, too, are showing interest in the relationship between antisocial behaviour and poor diet. At Stanislaus County Juvenile Hall, a detention centre for 3000 juveniles in Northern California, researchers modified the diets of all inmates over a two-year period. Junk food was banned and, instead, the facility's staff prepared nutritious snacks and treats which did not contain as much sugar or food additives. Snacks such as popcorn and unsweetened orange juice were also substituted for candy bars and soft drinks. The results showed that the incidence of serious antisocial behaviour declined by 21 per cent, assaults and fights declined by 25 per cent, and there were also reductions in suicide attempts, verbal threats and disobedience.[100]

Another remarkable study carried out among young offenders in a similar institution found that, on average, displays of antisocial behaviour could be cut by about 50 per cent simply by reducing their sugar consumption. The researchers replaced soft drinks and junk food snacks with fruit juices and nutritional snacks, and eliminated high-sugar desserts and cereals. After 12 months, the number of assaults had been lowered by 82 per cent, thefts had been cut by 77 per cent, general rule violations were reduced by 23 per cent, and fighting was diminished by 13 per cent. Most significantly, after the experiment ended and the inmates were allowed to eat junk food again, it was found that incidents of antisocial behaviour once again climbed to their previous levels.[101]

The one-week diet

If you suspect that your child's hyperactivity is related to a food allergy, try the one-week diet. This is based on the idea that hyperactive behaviour – if it is caused by an allergy to a foodstuff – will disappear while your child is eating a plain diet, and return when the offending food is reintroduced.

This diet requires attention to detail, diligence and accurate recording, but it is definitely worth trying. So for the first week make sure your child doesn't eat any of the following seven foods, which are thought to be the most likely to produce an allergic reaction:

- Milk
- Wheat
- Egg
- Cocoa
- Sugar
- Corn
- Food colourings

It's not going to be very easy for you, because many of these substances are present in much of our diet. But stick at it – just for a week, at least.

After one week without any of these suspect seven foods, see if there's an improvement. If there is, you're on the way to discovering what causes your child to be hyperactive, and to curing the problem too. So during the second week reintroduce them, one by one:

- Sunday – milk (dairy products, cheese, yogurt)
- Monday – wheat (bread, cake, bakery stuffs)
- Tuesday – sugar
- Wednesday – egg
- Thursday – cocoa (chocolate)
- Friday – food colouring (observe labelling)
- Saturday – corn

Should you discover a food affecting your child's hyperactivity, alter his or her diet permanently to eliminate the offending foodstuff.

LifePoints Power Foods: Immune Deficiency

Maintaining a healthy immune system should be a top priority for all of us, because without it we are – quite literally – dead. Your immune system is the crucial means by which your body resists disease and infection; it is also a defence system you almost certainly know little about and take completely for granted. And yet there has never been a more important time than now for you to take action to bolster your body's natural defences, because every day you are exposed to an ever-increasing bombardment of pollutants, toxins, bacteria and stress which, collectively, can weaken or destroy your health. Conventional medicine has focused first on understanding, then on replicating, the work of the immune system using drugs. But this is not the only way to fight infection. Alternative medicine has, for centuries, used natural substances specifically to boost the body's own immune system – not to replace it. And recently, mounting scientific research confirms that many of these older, natural remedies are indeed effective. We believe that it is better to have a strong natural immunity to disease than to rely on drugs to cure you after you've succumbed to illness. So here we present you with a unique collection of little-known measures which have been proven to protect and fortify your body's own immune system.

You and your body function, health-wise, in a hostile universe comprising a teeming ocean of viruses, bacteria, cancers, pollen, mould spores and man-made chemicals and pollutants. Collectively these are all known as *antigens*. Sometimes it seems a miracle that the body survives at all in such a potentially harmful environment! That it does so is down to the strength and durability of your immune system.

When your body comes under attack from these antigens it is your immune system which comes to its rescue and fights back. Your immune system is organically programmed to respond in a flexible and adaptable manner to ward off the potentially invasive antigens which can make you fall victim to illness. It does this in a host of complex ways, some of which are still not fully understood. But to put it simply, the human immune system functions in two broad ways. First, it can produce substances known as antibodies in response to invading antigens. Antibodies circulate in the blood and other body fluids, and when they find an antigen they try to neutralize it. Second, the body's immune response can also activate cells known as macrophages, which destroy invading micro-organisms by engulfing and digesting them. This second variety of immune response characteristically produces a raised red area on the skin in response to an infection. Antibodies are produced by white blood cells which originate in the bone marrow, and macrophages are stimulated by white blood cells which originate in the thymus gland. Obviously, any disease which affects the bone marrow or thymus can have very serious effects on the entire immune system.

Your basic defensive strategy

Some simple dietary measures can help to boost your immune system, fight potential immune deficiency and build resistance to illness. First, some general points:

- There is evidence that sugar (and this includes table sugar, fruit juices and honey) can suppress the functioning of the immune system.[102] So reduce your sugar consumption.
- Alcohol depresses your immune function, and it can also prevent your body from absorbing vital nutrients from food. There is no question that chronic alcoholics suffer from a depressed immune system.[103] What is not so clear – yet – is just how much 'ordinary' social drinking affects your long-term immunity. One study from France looked at the way the human immune system functioned before, during and after drinking a large whisky, and concluded that alcohol consumption had only a 'limited effect' on immune function.[104] But even this study revealed some short-term immune depression. The prudent conclusion is that you should restrict alcohol consumption to the occasional social drink and eliminate it when your immune system is particularly vulnerable or run-down.
- Short-term fasting can help to boost your immune system when it is under attack (for example, when you've got a cold coming on). Studies show that fasting for up to 36 hours can

increase the number of active phagocytes (which form the first line of defence against infection) in your body by up to 50 per cent.[105] But don't go beyond this time limit when you're ill, otherwise your immune system may not be able to cope.

- A good intake of protein is essential for a strong immune system. People always think of 'meat' as being the only source of protein, but from the health point of view meat has some serious drawbacks. Indisputable scientific evidence shows that meat-eaters consistently suffer from more serious illness than non-meat-eaters (cancers, heart disease, etc.).[106] So make sure you're getting several good plant food sources of protein – among the best is the soya bean and all its associated products.

- Since you should be particularly looking to eat meals rich in vitamins and minerals, this means avoiding processed and refined foodstuffs generally. Retrain your appetite to desire a bowl full of luscious salad instead of overprocessed food such as white sugar, white rice, white flour, and the cakes, pastries, bread, rolls and pies that are made from them. Instead, turn to complex carbohydrates such as whole grains, wholewheat pastas and wholegrain breads.

Vitamin B6 foods

A number of studies have shown that a low level of vitamin B6 (sometimes known as pyridoxine) in the body is connected to a generally weakened immune system, and some studies have even linked a deficiency in this vitamin to the development of cancer.[107] Additionally, several more studies have shown that high doses of B6 can suppress cancerous tumour growth.[108] Since it is well known that this vitamin plays a vital role in many physiological processes, such as amino acid metabolism, lipid metabolism and, of course, in the immune system itself, some scientists believe that a great many people could be suffering from 'subclinical' B6 deficiency and that this may have an important part to play in the development of diseases such as atherosclerosis, multiple sclerosis and other degenerative diseases of the central nervous system.[109] Other studies have shown that B6 supplementation in elderly people can be an effective way to stimulate and improve the functioning of their immunity to disease.[110] Vitamin B6 is stored mainly in the liver, and an average adult will, at any one time, have about 16–27mg stored in their body.[111] However, since B6 is a water-soluble vitamin it is regularly excreted from the body, meaning that we all need to provide ourselves with a continuous intake. Foods such as oat bran and oat germ, hummus, avocados, bananas, brewers' yeast, yeast extract, brown rice, parsley and spinach all contain useful amounts of it.

Vitamin E foods

The primary role of vitamin E is to protect the body tissues from oxygen damage. But, in addition to this, vitamin E is a very important nutrient for the optimal functioning of the immune system. It has been shown experimentally that when diets are lacking in vitamin E the immune response is depressed. Correspondingly, when diets are supplemented with levels of vitamin E that are rather higher than those considered to be nutritionally 'adequate', the immune response is likewise enhanced.[112] Many of us today consume considerable amounts of polyunsaturated fatty acids, because we correctly believe that this is a healthier alternative than eating saturated animal fats. However, there is in fact evidence to suggest that high levels of polyunsaturated fatty acids may reduce the effective functioning of the immune system. An intake of vitamin E can act to overcome this immunosuppression.[113] The richest dietary sources of vitamin E are seed oils and nuts, whole grains, leafy green vegetables and eggs. Wheat germ oil is a particularly rich source.

Vitamin C foods

It has been proven experimentally that high levels of vitamin C can protect tissue levels of vitamin E and may well contribute to the strengthening of the immune system that vitamin E brings about.[114] This is how specialist Dr Stuart Berger of New York puts it:

> The major factor in your immune system – the white blood cells – has a lot of housekeeping chores to do; which includes isolating and destroying bad viruses and bacteria. The white blood cells cannot do this without the help of vitamin C. Vitamins help to neutralize toxins in your body –

especially that overload of toxins that occur when you are sick.[115]

Despite continuing controversy over the claims made for vitamin C, there is a body of evidence which indicates that it does indeed play an important part in strengthening and maintaining a healthy immune system.[116] Researchers in Belgium discovered that 500mg of vitamin C administered daily (through intramuscular injection) for one month significantly bolstered the immune system in a group of healthy volunteers over 70. The researchers concluded that vitamin C should be considered a 'successful, non-toxic and inexpensive means of improving the immunity'.[117]

Beta-carotene foods

Beta-carotene is a pre-vitamin A compound found in plants, and which is converted inside the body to vitamin A. Beta-carotene has been shown to have immuno-stimulatory powers. In one study, eleven HIV-positive patients were given 30mg per day of beta-carotene for four months. All of them showed greater immune system activity after treatment.[118] Beta-carotene is freely available in foods such as broccoli, tomatoes, carrots, sweet potatoes, parsnips, squash, beets, spinach, and fruits like cantaloupes and papayas. Other rich sources of beta-carotene are easy to spot: bright green, orange or yellow fruits or vegetables almost always contain useful amounts.

Zinc

This mineral has been found to aid the healing of wounds and is crucial to proper immune cell function. A low zinc level can impair your immune response and so make you susceptible to many infectious diseases.[119] In-depth studies have shown that lack of zinc is a major nutritional deficiency in many developed countries. The recommended daily allowances for zinc range from 5–10mg for children to 12–15mg for adults (breast-feeding women need 16–19mg daily). However, the zinc content of the average diet is between 10 and 15mg per day, thus putting millions of people below the recommended level.[120] The elderly consume an average of only 7–10mg per day. Researchers from the National Research Council on AIDS in Italy believe that zinc supplements may enhance the immune system of people with AIDS because the mineral is involved in maintaining high levels of thymulin, which is a hormone from the thymus gland that regulates immune response.[121] People with AIDS often have a low level of zinc.

Selenium foods

The human body needs tiny amounts of this trace element. One study has shown that a concentration of 0.7 parts per million in the body can increase antibody production by seven times.[122] And with a concentration of 2.8 parts per million, antibody production shot up 30 times! It has been known for 30 years that selenium is essential and vital to life, even though needed in only fantastically small quantities. But it is only recently – with the surge of deaths from cancers and AIDS – that serious attention has once again focused on selenium. The most minute trace amounts of selenium have a 'synergistic' effect on vitamin E; in other words, it works with vitamin E in the body to strengthen your immune response.

In America, the National Research Council has recommended a daily intake of 50–200mcg of selenium for adults (a microgram is one-thousandth of a milligram, so 200mcg equals 0.2mg). However, one authority – Gerhard Schrauzer, PhD, of the University of California – believes that 250–300mcg can protect against most cancers, and that most people consume only about 100mcg daily.[123] At higher doses, selenium can be toxic to the human body. Although it is not certain at precisely what level selenium begins to cause adverse effects, it has been found that doses of 900mcg (0.9mg) per day can make hair and nails fall out and can affect the nervous system.[124] You'd be unlikely to get this much from your diet, and supplements are clearly marked with the dosage they contain.

Uncommon weapons for your armoury

Conventional medicine is often very slow to consider the effectiveness of traditional medicines – sometimes, it seems as if the older remedies are deliberately overlooked in favour of the more exciting, but also more expensive, new drugs. The irony is, of course, that many drug developments are themselves based upon traditional folk and plant pharmaceutical preparations. So here are some of the more overlooked substances which you may wish to consider. It is always advisable to have the assistance of a qualified herbalist or other practitioner when deciding on treatment and dosages.

- Purple cornflower (*Echinaceae angustifolia*, also *Echinaceae purpurea*). This plant produces rich purple flowers, and was originally used by Native Americans as a blood purifier and snake bite remedy. It is now cultivated in Britain and elsewhere. The dried root is used to prepare a liquid extract. It has been shown to stimulate macrophage cells, which seek out and destroy invading bacteria and viruses.[125] The suggested dose is 0.5–1 drachm of the liquid extract (a drachm is an apothecary's measure, approximately 3.8879g.[126]

- Goldenseal (*Hydrastis canadensis*) was also discovered by Native Americans, who valued the root for its medicinal properties and used the yellow stain from the rest of the plant as a dye for clothes and faces. Goldenseal root contains approximately 4 per cent of an alkaloid called berberine, which is the main active ingredient of the plant (and is very poisonous if the prescribed dose is exceeded). Berberine has been proven to be a powerful stimulator of macrophage activity.[127]

- Liquorice (*Glycyrrhiza glabra*) is so well known to most people that it needs no introduction. However, the liquorice most of us are familiar with is the rather sickly flavouring found in children's sweets. By this stage in the manufacturing process, it has no useful medicinal activity left. Medicinal use of liquorice root was first recorded in the third century BC by the Greeks, who used it to treat asthma, dry cough and all diseases of the chest; since then it has a long history both as a food flavouring and as a medicinal ingredient. Recent research has shown that some of the active ingredients in liquorice root can actually increase the production of interferon. (Interferon is a protein which is produced by cells when they are invaded by viruses. When released into the bloodstream, it acts as a messenger to instruct healthy cells to manufacture an enzyme that counters the infection.)[128] In the laboratory, liquorice has also been shown to inhibit the growth of viruses such as herpes simplex,[129] and it has also been shown to act against a number of common bacteria (including streptococcus) and *Candida albicans*.[130]

- Consider taking spirulina, which provides a wide range of nutrients. Chlorella is a similar edible algae, which also provides a broad-spectrum mega-dose of natural nutrients to bolster the immune system in multiple ways.

- Many people find a macrobiotic diet to be very effective in helping to enhance the immune response. One specialist, Dr J. D. Kaiser, who practises medicine in San Francisco, recommends a 'modified macrobiotic' diet for the treatment of people with AIDS, including fruits, vegetables, wholewheat pasta, whole grains, shiitake mushrooms. Garlic, ginger, olive and sesame oil are recommended; sugar, alcohol and caffeine are not.[132] Says Dr Kaiser: 'I believe that we stand today on the cutting edge of using natural therapies as a means of treating many medical conditions that to this point have been poorly managed by standard medical therapies alone.'

- Germanium has been shown to induce production of interferon, enhance normal killer-cell activity and activate macrophages in laboratory studies. Dr Stephen A. Levine, PhD, writing in the *Journal of Orthomolecular Medicine*, states that organic germanium has demonstrated marked anti-tumour effects, as well as interferon-inducing activity. It has also restored immune function in immune-depressed animals. According to Dr Levine, 'These immunostimulant effects were achieved with oral doses, and no harmful side-effects were noted'.[133]

- Garlic has been shown to improve the natural killer-cell activity in people with AIDS. Garlic is thought to be a particularly valuable tool for reviving the immune system because it is one of the richest sources of organic selenium and germanium. It also contains magnesium, 17 amino acids and vitamins B1, A and C.

In one study, 10 AIDS patients were given garlic extracts as a food supplement for 12 weeks. A 5g dose of the extract was taken daily during the first six weeks, and a 10g dose was taken each day for the second six weeks. During the experimental period, three patients experienced gastrointestinal and neurological problems and were unable to take the supplement (they later died). All the seven patients who were fit enough to take the supplement showed signs of a strengthening immune system. They reported fewer bouts of diarrhoea, genital herpes, candidiasis and pansinusitis with recurrent fever.[134]

- The following natural medicines have been used by Japanese nutritionists to stimulate a jaded immune system. Many of these substances, although very familiar to oriental cooks, are largely unknown in the West and untested by Western science. However, some good scientific news does surface from time to time. For example, it is now established beyond doubt that Japanese green tea has anti-tumour properties. Researchers from the National Cancer Research Institute in Tokyo discovered that fewer people die from cancer in the Shizouka area of Japan than in other regions. Shizouka produces much of Japan's green tea, and the locals drink it in large quantities. After isolating one of its active ingredients (epigallocatechin gallate, or EGCG), they discovered that EGCG can indeed block tumour activity.[135] Unfortunately, this applies only to green tea which contains sizeable quantities of EGCG – ordinary British tea contains virtually none. Here are some other substances which, one day, we hope may prove to be equally useful: LEM (Lentinus Edodes Mycelia, an extract from the shiitake mushroom), hijiki (a sea vegetable), iwanori (a sea vegetable), beer yeast, yogurt, natto beans (fermented soya beans), wild taro (a type of starchy potato), umeboshi (salt pickled plum), kumquat (a fruit), jujube, pine seeds.

LIFEPOINTS POWER FOODS: INSOMNIA

Insomnia is a pattern of either waking repeatedly during the night or having persistent difficulty in falling asleep in the first place. For some people insomnia is a temporary affliction, passing within days or weeks; but for others it is a seemingly permanent part of their lives. Most people who suffer from insomnia would agree that it is an unpleasant and frustrating predicament, often driving them to despair and to a bottle of sedatives.

The cause of insomnia is usually psychological. It has always been associated with depression, anxiety and general stress, so if you suffer from insomnia you will probably benefit from learning a relaxation technique. Nevertheless, all insomniacs should take a good look at their diet to see whether they are eating something which could be the cause of their sleeplessness, or whether they are failing to eat something which might help them sleep.

- Sleeplessness in children usually means sleeplessness in parents, too! Recent research from Belgium[136] has revealed that a previously undiagnosed intolerance to cow's milk may be a cause of insomnia in children. In the Belgian studies, once the children had milk eliminated from their diet their sleeping problems dramatically improved. An intolerance to cow's milk is also common in adults, so try eliminating all dairy products from your diet – and that of your children.

- Tryptophan is an essential amino acid which is synthesized into serotonin, a compound in your brain which can initiate sleep. Nuts such as peanuts, pecans, walnuts and brazil nuts all contain tryptophan and a snack of these before retiring may help you fall asleep. A serving of baked beans is also effective.

- Increase your intake of the B group of vitamins. These vitamins help your body to cope with stress, a common cause of insomnia. The B vitamins are essential to the proper functioning of your nervous system and influence your moods and your emotional wellbeing. Foods rich in the B vitamins are brewers' yeast, nuts and seeds and all whole grains.

- You might think a nightcap will help you conquer your insomnia, and it might work once. However, alcohol is one of many dietary factors which can actually inhibit sleep. Reduce your intake of alcohol and avoid a nightcap altogether. Coffee, chocolate, tea and many other drugs (such as marijuana and certain prescription drugs) also inhibit sleep and should be avoided.

- Reduce your intake of refined sugar as it can cause large fluctuations in your blood sugar level. Wakefulness at night is often caused by a sudden drop in your blood sugar level. Eat an evening meal low in sugar but high in complex carbohydrates to correct a tendency to wake, perhaps feeling hungry, in the middle of the night. Complex carbohydrates are

unprocessed grains, legumes and vegetables.
- A hot cup of camomile, hop or lemon verbena herbal tea has relaxing properties and makes a good bedtime drink. Serve with a slice of lemon and a piece of cinnamon to make it really special.

LifePoints Power Foods: Migraine

We all have headaches from time to time, and when we do we often have a good idea of their cause – too much to drink the night before, eyestrain from working in a badly lit environment or the prospect of an unpleasant event in our lives, to name but three. But migraines are different. For a start, it is often difficult to pinpoint their cause, and their severity and duration, as any sufferer will tell you, can be quite awesome. Headaches are generally divided into two categories: tension headaches and vascular headaches. A tension headache is caused by muscle spasms in the neck and head, and is by far the most common form (about 90 per cent of headaches are thought to fall into this category). Tension headaches, which continue on and off for years, are often associated with chronic depression or some other emotional problem and are sometimes effectively treated by psychotherapy or relaxation training. Vascular headaches, however, are something different again. A migraine is a typical vascular headache; the symptoms may include a severe throbbing pain, often just on one side of the head, vertigo, visual disturbances, nausea and vomiting, and the attack may last a day or more. Basically, what seems to be happening is that blood vessels inside the head are dilating, so stimulating and causing pain to the membranous linings of the brain. Conventional therapy often includes treatment by vasoconstrictive drugs, which attempt to reduce the swelling of these blood vessels.

Whilst prescription medicines can sometimes solve the immediate problem of a migraine attack, none of them treats the underlying cause. So the sensible way to fight a migraine is on two fronts: first, try to prevent it from happening; and, second, conquer it when it does!

Prevent

The evidence shows that migraines are frequently triggered by certain foods, so this is a good starting point. If you are a sufferer, you may already suspect which foods are liable to bring on an attack. If not, follow this plan to identify the culprit.

First, make arrangements to eat a simple 'elimination' diet for several days – up to a week if you can. This should consist only of those foods which are least likely to cause an allergic reaction, such as:

- Brown rice
- Rice flour
- Puffed rice
- Cooked fruits (not citrus)
- Simple cooked vegetables (potatoes, cabbage, broccoli, etc.).

It should definitely *exclude* these foods, which experience shows are most likely to provoke an attack:

- Cheese
- Chocolate
- Red wine
- Wheat
- Corn
- Eggs
- Milk
- Shellfish
- Citrus fruits
- Coffee
- Tomatoes
- Strawberries.

If you feel better after your elimination diet, and haven't had an attack, that is a promising indication that food allergy may indeed be responsible for your attacks. To confirm this, reintroduce each one of the suspect foods into your diet every two days. At the first sign of an attack, you've found one of the culprits! This process sounds easy, but it actually requires a considerable amount of dedication to make it work. It is a painstaking procedure, but the rewards, if your detective work succeeds, will be worth it. A study published in the *Lancet* has established that 93 per cent of long-term sufferers can obtain relief by eliminating offending foods from their diet.[137] So give it a try!

And conquer!

Even if your migraine is not directly triggered by a specific food, diet can still be an important factor.

- At the University of Missouri, research has shown that people who suffer from migraine frequently suffer from hypoglycaemia as well.[138] Hypoglycaemia, or low blood sugar, has associated with it a wide-ranging list of other symptoms, including fatigue, irritability, indigestion, breathlessness and blurred vision. The condition can be diagnosed with a glucose-tolerance test which identifies any abnormal over-reaction to glucose. An overreaction brings about a severe drop in the blood sugar level and symptomatic headaches or migraine can result. People who have been identified as suffering from this condition have also been shown to have a magnesium deficiency. If you are a migraine sufferer, try including more magnesium-rich foods in your diet, preferably from organic sources. Magnesium is found in fresh green vegetables, whole grains, nuts and yeast extracts.

- Probably the most interesting dietary remedy for migraine is the common herb feverfew, which has been used to treat headaches since early Roman times. Several very exciting recent studies have proven that feverfew can indeed prevent migraine attacks.[139] One study found that 70 per cent of the people who consumed two or three fresh leaves of the bitter-tasting plant each day had fewer and less severe attacks than a comparable group of migraine sufferers who didn't use the plant.[140] Just how feverfew works is not clear – it contains sesquiterpene lactones – substances which are known to inhibit the release of the brain chemical called serotonin, thought to be one of the precipitating factors of migraine attacks. Be aware, however, that taking any drug, including feverfew, for a long time might lead to side-effects – so talk to your practitioner before embarking on treatment.

- Another foodstuff with possible anti-migraine effects is cayenne pepper. It contains an ingredient, capsaicin, which might be able to prevent and control migraine attacks by inhibiting platelet aggregation, one of the biological changes which may underlie attacks.[141]

- It is also possible that certain bacteria active in the colon may produce substances which produce an allergic migraine reaction in sensitive people. A course of colonic irrigation could therefore be of help.

LIFEPOINTS POWER FOODS: MULTIPLE SCLEROSIS

Multiple sclerosis (MS) is a degenerative disease of the central nervous system. In the course of the disease, myelin (which is a white, fatty substance that acts as an electrical insulator for the nerves) is progressively destroyed, and the formation of hard scar tissue on the protective myelin sheath which surrounds nerves stops the nerve cells from working. This scarring results in permanent loss of nervous control to areas of the body. MS is a crippling disease which attacks every body function; and with time it can be fatal. It affects both men and women, usually first being diagnosed between the ages of 20 and 40.

Literally dozens of causes have been suggested over the years. A great deal of research has gone into investigating the possibility that MS is caused by a virus, although to date it has not proved possible to pinpoint precisely which one. Similarly, it has long been suspected that MS is an autoimmune disease, a sort of allergic reaction in which the body responds to an antigen by acting against itself. Again, pinpointing the antigen in question has proved very difficult. Another theory proposes that giving cow's milk to infants predisposes them to nervous system injury later in life, because cow's milk has only one-fifth as much linoleic acid (an essentially fatty acid) as human breast milk, and linoleic acid makes up the building blocks for nervous tissues.[142] The list could go on and on. But while waiting for conclusive proof of cause it is possible to deal with multiple sclerosis so as to minimize its crippling effect and, perhaps, prolong life.

Diet and MS

Most health professionals have traditionally dismissed the idea that the cause of multiple sclerosis might be linked to diet. However, Dr Roy Swank, former Professor of Neurology at the University of Oregon, was intrigued by some wartime research. During World War II, the consumption of animal fat decreased in Western Europe. Meat and dairy products were rationed and, instead, consumption of grains and vegetables increased. It was noticed at this time that patients with MS had between two and two and a half times fewer hospitalizations during the war years, when saturated fat consumption was low.[143] Greatly excited by the possible implication of these findings, Dr Swank began treating his own patients with a low-fat diet. Over the next 35 years, he treated thousands of MS patients in this way. By any medical standard his results have been remarkable: patients' conditions improved by as much as 95 per cent.[144] Patients fared better if they had detected the disease early and had had few attacks, but even long-time MS sufferers experienced a slowdown in the disease's progression. The basics of his diet are:

- No more than 10g saturated fat per day
- 40–50g polyunsaturated fat (but *not* margarine or other hydrogenated fats)
- At least 1 teaspoon of cod liver oil daily
- Fish three times per week, other animal foods cut out.[145]

Protein intake should be kept up with a good supply of mixed vegetable proteins. The long-term results of the Swank diet show that of those who ate less than 20g of fat per day, only 31 per cent have died (close to normal) and the condition of the rest has deteriorated only slightly. Of those who ate more than 20g, 81 per cent have died.[146] [147] [148] However, many orthodox medical practitioners are still very wary of accepting such evidence. As an editorial in the medical magazine the *Lancet* stated:

> There are still no firm answers as to whether a relationship [between MS and dietary fats] does indeed exist and if so, what its mechanism might be . . . more work is needed at the biochemical level . . . Until such studies are undertaken, the rôle of lipids in MS cannot be said to be proven.[149]

But in the words of another doctor who uses the Swank diet to treat patients: 'I've been very gratified by the results of this dietary treatment, not only because the progress of most of my MS patients' disease has been halted, but also because their overall health has unquestionably improved.'[150]

LifePoints Power Foods: Osteoporosis

If you are a woman, by the time you are 60 there is a one in four chance that osteoporosis will have caused you to break a bone.[151] And more than 10 per cent of people who suffer a hip fracture caused by osteoporosis will die.[152] Osteoporosis literally means 'porous bones'. You may not even realize that you suffer from it until you suddenly break a bone – by which time the harm has been done. Other telltale signs can include severe back pain, loss of height or deformities such as a curvature of the spine. It is estimated that more than 50,000 women fracture their hip each year due to osteoporosis.[153] And the number of deaths from fractured hips is greater than the number of deaths from cancers of the cervix, uterus and breast combined,[154] which makes osteoporosis one of the major killers of our time.

Osteoporosis is caused by a slow loss of bone mass. By the age of 35 or so, your bones will be as strong as they're ever likely to be. The rest, as they say, is all downhill! Hormones in our bodies are responsible for continuously balancing the growth of new bone with the reabsorption of old bone. When levels of these hormones fall significantly, as happens in menopause, this balance is lost and a gradual loss of bone mass occurs. Eventually, the bones can become very brittle and break easily. In some women this process is sufficiently slow to avoid fractures, pain and loss of height. In others, however, the loss is rapid – some women can lose up to half of their bone mass within ten or so years of menopause, leaving them very vulnerable to easy fracture. Since it is clear that oestrogen, the female sex hormone, plays a protective role in the maintenance of bone mass, one current treatment for women suffering from osteoporosis is Hormone Replacement Therapy (HRT).

Unlike some modern-day epidemics, osteoporosis is not an equal opportunities disease. It discriminates on the grounds of gender, race and age. Both men and women *can* suffer from osteoporosis, but it is rarer in men (one estimate is that only one in 40 men is ever diagnosed as having it).[155] Oriental and Caucasian women are most at risk due to their tendency to have thinner, lighter bones. Women of African, Mediterranean or Aboriginal extraction are less likely to suffer from osteoporosis.

Hormone Replacement Therapy

HRT provides your body with a supplement of the female hormone oestrogen. While every last detail of the mechanism by which oestrogen slows down bone loss is not yet known, doctors have known about its usefulness in treating this complaint for over 50 years,[156] and there is no doubt that it works. HRT has a number of very worthwhile advantages:

- It slows down the loss of bone mineral content, so decreasing the likelihood of fractures of the spine, hips and wrists.
- It prevents loss of height.
- It lowers LDL cholesterol in your blood and increases HDL cholesterol, thus prolonging life expectancy by decreasing the risk of heart disease.
- It decreases the incidence of hot flushes.
- It decreases the risk of ovarian cancer.[157]

On the other hand, concerns have been expressed about its long-term safety (as they have for the oestrogen-based contraceptive pill). Although many women – and some doctors – are concerned about an increased risk of cancer from HRT, most of the scientific evidence does not confirm these worries. While some scientific studies do indeed show that oestrogen therapy may increase the risk of developing cancer,[158] today's HRT includes other hormones (progestogens) which studies show can actually reduce the cancer risk quite appreciably.[159] [160] This is an area of ongoing research, and it is worth keeping up to date with the latest findings. There are, however, some problems associated with HRT, as with all drugs. These can sometimes include breast soreness, gallstones, weight gain, return of periods and breakthrough bleeding. You should obviously discuss these and other aspects of HRT with your doctor before commencing treatment.

How to battle brittle bones

Treating osteoporosis successfully is one thing, but preventing it is even better. Here are some simple changes you can make to your lifestyle which can slow the rate of bone loss and, if started at a young enough age, prevent osteoporosis from developing in the first place. The potential for suffering from osteoporosis is now thought to be laid down in childhood. So if you have a daughter, begin now to instil in her the importance of following this four-point prevention programme:

1 Make exercise part of your way of life

Especially important are forms of exercise that are weight-bearing such as walking, dancing, running and many sports. Swimming and chess playing, for instance, are *not* weight-bearing exercises. Proper exercise exerts the muscles around your bones, stimulating them to maintain bone density. Leading a sedentary life will increase the likelihood of osteoporosis developing later in your life.

2 Avoid smoking, caffeine and excess alcohol

- Smoking can increase your risk of suffering from osteoporosis.[161]
- Caffeine is found in tea, coffee and chocolate. A study of women aged 36 to 45 found that those who drank two cups of coffee a day suffered a net calcium loss of 22mg daily. One cup meant a loss of just 6mg daily. The authors concluded that negative calcium balance of 40mg per day (i.e. about four cups) was enough to explain the 1 to 1.5 per cent loss in skeletal mass in postmenopausal women each year.[162] So cut down your caffeine consumption.
- Alcohol, except in moderation, speeds bone loss because it interferes with the way your body absorbs calcium. If you are a woman, keep within the 14 units per week recommendation (this figure is for health purposes only; it has nothing to do with drink-driving regulations).

3 Get regular doses of sunlight

Sunlight reacts with a substance in your skin – dehydrocholesterol – to produce vitamin D. This vitamin is essential for the proper absorption of calcium and a deficiency will cause you to lose bone mass. Most people get enough vitamin D just by being outside for part of the day with their face, hands and arms exposed.[163] If you don't get out regularly, you may need to eat food which is fortified with it.

4 Choose the right food

When selecting foods, you need to take into consideration the effects of calcium, magnesium and boron.

● **Calcium** The UK recommended daily allowance of calcium for adults is currently 500mg per day, and the American one is 800mg. Yet a consensus at a recent conference on osteoporosis in Virginia, USA, put the recommended level as high as 1500mg per day for women,[164] and another experimental study shows that about 1200mg per day is the right level to keep the body in calcium balance.[165] So how much calcium do you actually need? Obviously, different people will need different amounts. At a symposium organized by the National Osteoporosis Society, Dr Chris Robinson, a lecturer at Newcastle-upon-Tyne Medical School, outlined the following requirements:

Age/Condition	Intake requirement (mg)
Normal adult	800
Adolescent growth	1100
Pregnancy	1000
Lactation	1200
Elderly with HRT	1000
Elderly without HRT	1500

However, 1500mg is nearly ½ lb of hard cheese, four cups of yogurt or five cups of milk a day! Most people would find it difficult to include these amounts of dairy foods in their diet, and in any case there are undesirable health implications in eating such quantities of these foods.

Dairy foods tend to be very high in fat, especially saturated fat, and cholesterol. Regular consumption of such large amounts would increase the risk of obesity, cardiovascular disease and stroke. If you wish to eat dairy foods, choose those with reduced fat content.

Consuming large amounts of animal protein is undesirable for a number of reasons. When scientists from Andrews University, Michigan, studied the bone mass (by direct photon absorptiometry) of 1600 women living in southwestern Michigan they found some surprising results. Women who had eaten a vegetarian diet for at least 20 years had lost an average of only 18 per cent of their bone mineral by the time they were 80. On the other hand, women who did not eat a vegetarian diet had lost an average of 35 per cent of their bone mineral. Interestingly, there was no statistical difference in the nutrient intakes between the two groups.[166] The difference in bone loss could be explained by the different type of protein consumed. A diet high in animal-based proteins increases the amount of acid in the body. This triggers a buffering mechanism, which releases stored calcium from the bones. The body would normally reabsorb the calcium released, but the animal protein inhibits the parathyroid function that orders this reabsorption. The body then excretes the calcium, causing bone loss. One researcher who put this theory to the test concluded: 'This study suggests that a diet higher in vegetable protein might actually be somewhat protective against osteoporosis.'[167]

So how can you take in enough calcium to protect yourself from osteoporosis without consuming excessive quantities of animal-based foodstuffs? Non-meat foods rich in calcium include:

- Dairy products (low RiskPoints, please!)
- Tofu
- Sesame seeds and paste (tahini)
- Pumpkin and sunflower seeds
- Molasses
- Carob
- Dried figs, currants and apricots
- Almond and brazil nuts
- Porridge
- Spinach, seaweed and other green leafy vegetables.

● **Magnesium** This mineral works with other vitamins and minerals, including calcium, to promote bone growth and the healthy functioning of nerves and muscle tissue. A deficiency in magnesium can affect the manufacture of vitamin D, so magnesium is important in preventing osteoporosis. Magnesium is a constituent of chlorophyll and so is abundant in green vegetables. Other excellent sources are whole grains, wheat germ, molasses, seeds and nuts, apples and figs.

● **Boron** This trace mineral helps to prevent calcium loss and subsequent loss of bone mass. It is also thought to help in the manufacture of vitamin D in the body. The first study ever to look at the nutritional effects of boron in humans took place in 1987. Twelve postmenopausal women were fed a diet very low in boron for 17 weeks, after which they were given a daily supplement of 3mg for a further seven weeks. The addition of boron had a dramatic effect – the women lost 40 per cent less calcium and 30 per cent less magnesium through their urine. The study therefore concluded that boron can reduce bodily losses of elements necessary to maintain bone integrity and to prevent osteoporosis. What was even more exciting was the discovery that the boron supplement could double the most active form of oestrogen (estradiol 17B) in the blood of the women – their estradiol levels equalled those of women on oestrogen replacement therapy. Curtiss Hunt, of the US Human Nutrition Research Center, said he 'suspects the body needs boron to synthesize oestrogen, vitamin D and other steroid hormones. And it may protect these hormones against rapid breakdown.'[168]

Foods rich in boron are easily obtained; they include apples, grapes, pears, prunes, dates, raisins, almonds, peanuts and hazelnuts. This provides yet another good reason to include fresh food in your diet every day.

And finally . . .

The vitamin B complex and vitamin K are both thought to play a role in the prevention of osteoporosis. The B group vitamins are available in brewers' yeast, whole grains, molasses, nuts and seeds and dark green leafy vegetables. Vitamin K is present in cauliflower, soybeans, molasses, safflower oil and, again, dark green leafy vegetables.

Several commonly used drugs can induce significant calcium loss, particularly aluminium-containing antacids. If these antacids are used for prolonged periods of time they may produce bone abnormalities by interfering with calcium and phosphorus metabolism and so contribute to the development of osteoporosis.[169] If you want to use an antacid, choose one which does not include aluminium in its ingredients.

LifePoints Power Foods: Ulcers

Ulcers are sore-like flaws in the mucus-membrane lining of the upper digestive tract which leaves the lining vulnerable to damage from gastric juices and the digestive enzyme pepsin. The gastric, or stomach, ulcer and the duodenal ulcer are both forms of peptic ulcer – the duodenal ulcer is the more common and affects men more than women. The main symptom of an ulcer is upper-abdominal pain suffered about one hour after a meal or during the night. The development of an ulcer is usually associated with smoking, over-reliance on aspirin, food allergy or, in some people, stress.

To treat your ulcer and prevent recurrence, use this three-step plan:

1 Search and destroy

Identify those aspects of your lifestyle which are implicated in the development of your ulcer – then change them!

- One person's stress is another's holiday. You must decide whether the level of stress you live with is suited to you or not. If not, make a firm commitment to yourself to lower your stress level drastically.
- Monitor the drugs you take. Aspirin damages the lining of the stomach, and if you take it regularly you are simply inviting an ulcer to happen! Only take it when absolutely necessary, and investigate other forms of pain relief outlined in this book.
- Antacids are commonly taken to soothe the pain of an ulcer. However, there may be some unwanted side-effects which you should know about. For instance, antacids containing calcium carbonate can cause kidney stones; and others containing aluminium are suspected of contributing to a build-up of this metal in the brain.
- If you take other drugs on a regular basis, consult your doctor to ensure they are not complicating your ulcer problem; or look up the particular drug in the British National Formulary, available to purchase or at your local library.
- Stop smoking. Smoking seems seriously to complicate, maybe even cause, ulcer problems.
- Try an elimination diet to determine which food (or foods)

aggravates your ulcer. It is possible that some ulcers are a particularly painful form of allergic response. If you allow yourself two or three weeks to do the diet properly, you may well discover one or two culprits which you can then exclude from your diet. Those most often excluded are milk, strong spices, garlic, onions, red meats, beer, cheese and chocolate.

2 Promote healing

- Continue to avoid smoking and the drugs, foods and levels of stress which you have addressed in Step 1.
- Eat your evening meal at least four hours before you go to bed. The level of acid in your stomach usually drops as your stomach empties; this precaution helps ensure you get a good, pain-free night's sleep.
- Drink hot beverages rather cooler than you normally would, certainly cooler than scalding temperature. Very hot drinks are suspected of damaging the lining of the stomach, and it has been shown that peptic ulcer sufferers have a tendency to prefer much hotter beverages than other people.[170]
- Drink 1 l (2 pints) of raw cabbage juice each day for seven to ten days. Researchers at Stanford University School of Medicine have discovered that it can have a profound healing effect on ulcers.[171] Try to prepare it yourself from organic cabbages, or buy one of the bottled organic cabbage juices available in health food shops.

3 Protect and prevent

Now begin to include substances in your diet which will actively improve the health of your intestines and perhaps prevent your ulcer from recurring.

- Avoid coffee, alcohol, tea and fried foods in addition to the food or foods you have eliminated from your diet.
- Eat foods rich in the vitamin B-complex. These include whole grains, legumes, molasses, brewers' yeast, nuts and seeds and green leafy vegetables. These foods help to counteract the effects of stress on the body, and studies have shown that patients with low levels of the B group of vitamins also have high levels of stomach acid.[172]
- Increase your intake of vitamins A and E. Both are fat-soluble

vitamins which benefit the health of the mucus membranes that line your stomach and duodenum. They are available in supplement form, but you can find them in your food, too. For vitamin A, eat dark yellow and dark green fruits and vegetables such as carrot, squash, pomegranate, spinach, broccoli, avocado. For vitamin E, eat cold-pressed vegetable oils, wheat germ, molasses and leafy vegetables.

- Zinc is a mineral which aids in digestion and promotes healing. It is available in supplement form, or you can eat foods rich in zinc such as pumpkin and sunflower seeds, mushrooms, soybeans and brewers' yeast.

- Amend your diet to include foods high in fibre. A high-fibre diet is known to improve intestinal health provided the food is well chewed. Select foods from the whole grain, beans and pulses, fresh fruit and vegetable groups to ensure an intake of approximately 40g of fibre per day.

PART EIGHT: THE LIFEPOINTS FOOD COUNTER AND LIFEPOINTS FOOD GROUPS

Using the Counter

The foods that follow have been categorized into the six Life-Points food groups (if a recipe, according to the major ingredient). This makes it easy for you to plan your day's diet, choosing the best food from each group. If, however, you want to check the LifePoints rating for one specific food, you'll find it quickest to use the index to locate it.

For your convenience, foods in the Counter are presented in common serving sizes. When a food might be consumed in several different serving sizes, we've given a choice of measures. Because of rounding down, most foods show zero RiskPoints and LifePoints at very small serving sizes (e.g. one teaspoon). Do not assume that you can simply scale this up massively (e.g. from one teaspoon to one cup) and still get away with zero RiskPoints!

Ideally, the serving size you actually consume should be as close as possible to that given here if you want the RiskPoints and LifePoints numbers to be really accurate. Here's a very useful tip: if the RiskPoints number of the food is low (i.e. in single digits), then the accuracy of the serving size is far less important. Let's illustrate this with two foods. First, let's say you choose a monster spear of broccoli, boiled or steamed. In the Counter, an average spear weighs 180g and yields 3 RiskPoints and 12 LifePoints; but your spear weighs 270g. Even though your serving size is 50 per cent greater than that listed, your RiskPoints will only go from 3 to 5 (rounded up), which is a trivial difference. But take another food – say, broccoli in cheese sauce, made with whole milk. The RiskPoints for a serving of 115g is a significant 37. If you increase the serving size of this dish by 50 per cent, your RiskPoints will go up to 55. So the greater the RiskPoints in the food, the more important it is to be accurate about the serving size. If you do need to calculate new RiskPoints and LifePoints figures for a food because your serving size is different to ours, please remember that you will get maximum accuracy by working with the food weight in grams.

Spend as long as you can browsing through the following pages – you'll find the information and insights they contain quite remarkable! We suggest you put a mark beside any food which has a particularly good profile and which you'd like to include in your eating pattern at some future point.

Food	RiskPoints ✘	LifePoints ✔
Acerola: juice (1 fl. oz/30g)	0	6
Acerola: raw (1 fruit/5g)	0	1
Apple: baked with sugar, flesh and skin (1 fruit/138g)	0	2
Apple: boiled without skin (½ cup slices/86g)	0	0
Apple: canned, drained (½ cup slices/102g)	1	0
Apple: dehydrated (low-moisture) sulphured, stewed (½ cup/97g)	0	0
Apple: dehydrated (low-moisture) sulphured, uncooked (½ cup/30g)	0	1
Apple: dried sulphured, stewed (½ cup/128g)	0	1
Apple: dried sulphured, uncooked (½ cup/43g)	0	2
Apple: frozen, heated (½ cup slices/103g)	0	0
Apple: juice, canned or bottled, with added vitamin C (1 cup/248g)	0	3
Apple: juice, canned or bottled, without added vitamin C (1 cup/248g)	0	1
Apple: juice, from frozen concentrate, with added vitamin C (1 cup/239g)	0	2
Apple: juice, from frozen concentrate, without added vitamin C (1 cup/239g)	0	0
Apple: microwaved without skin (½ cup slices/85g)	0	0
Apple: raw with skin (1 fruit/138g)	1	1

	RiskPoints ✗	LifePoints ✔
Apple: raw without skin (1 fruit/128g)	0	1
Apple sauce: canned, with added vitamin C (½ cup/122g)	0	1
Apple sauce: canned, without added vitamin C (½ cup/122g)	0	1
Apricot: canned, in juice, with skin solids and liquid (1 cup halves/248g)	0	4
Apricot: dehydrated (low-moisture) sulphured, stewed (½ cup/124g)	0	6
Apricot: dehydrated (low-moisture) sulphured, uncooked (½ cup/60g)	0	8
Apricot: dried sulphured, stewed (½ cup halves/125g)	0	4
Apricot: dried sulphured, uncooked (½ cup halves/65g)	0	7
Apricot: juice, canned, with added vitamin C (1 cup/251g)	0	4
Apricot: juice, canned, without added vitamin C (1 cup/251g)	0	3
Apricot: raw (3 fruits/106g)	1	3
Avocado: raw (1 fruit/201g)	76	18
Avocado: raw (½ cup puree/115g)	38	9
Banana: dehydrated or banana powder (1 tbsp/6g)	0	0
Banana: raw (1 cup mashed/225g)	3	13
Banana: raw (1 fruit without skin/114g)	1	6
Blackberry: canned in syrup (½ cup/128g)	0	4
Blackberry: raw (½ cup/72g)	0	3

	RiskPoints ✗	LifePoints ✔
Blackberry: blackberry and apple, stewed (½ cup/72g)	0	1
Blackcurrant: raw (½ cup/56g)	0	2
Blackcurrant: stewed (½ cup/70g)	0	3
Blueberry: canned, in syrup (½ cup/128g)	1	1
Blueberry: frozen (½ cup/128g)	0	0
Blueberry: raw (½ cup/75g)	0	0
Boysenberry: canned, in syrup (½ cup/128g)	0	4
Boysenberry: frozen (½ cup/70g)	0	0
Breadfruit: raw (¼ small fruit/96g)	0	3
Bullock's-heart: see 'Custard-apple'		
Cape gooseberry: see 'Groundcherry'		
Carambola: raw (1 fruit without seeds/127g)	1	2
Carissa: raw (1 fruit without skin and seeds/20g)	0	0
Cherimoya: raw (½ fruit without skin and seeds/273g)	1	3
Cherry: pie filling (commercial) (½ cup/125g)	0	3
Cherry: sour, red, canned in syrup, solids and liquid (½ cup/126g)	0	2
Cherry: sour, red, frozen (1 cup unthawed/155g)	1	3
Cherry: sour, red, raw (1 cup with pits/103g)	0	2
Cherry: sweet, canned, in juice, solids and liquid (1 cup without pits/250g)	0	4

	RiskPoints ✘	LifePoints ✔
Cherry: sweet, raw (1 cup/145g)	3	3
Cherry: sweet, raw (10 fruits/68g)	1	1
Cherry: sweet, stewed (1 cup/250g)	0	2
Chinese date: *see* 'Jujube'		
Chinese gooseberry: *see* 'Kiwi fruit'		
Clementine: whole (1 fruit/100g)	0	3
Crabapple: raw (1 cup slices with skin/110g)	0	1
Cranberry: Cranberry-orange relish, canned (½ cup/138g)	0	1
Cranberry: juice cocktail, bottled (1 cup/253g)	0	2
Cranberry: raw (1 cup whole/95g)	0	1
Cranberry: sauce, canned, sweetened (½ cup/138g)	0	1
Currant: red and white, raw (½ cup/56g)	0	1
Currant: zante, dried (½ cup/72g)	0	6
Custard-apple: raw (100g)	1	3
Damson plums: raw (1 cup slices/165g)	0	4
Damson plums: raw (1 fruit/66g)	0	1
Damson plums: stewed (3 fruits/133g)	0	0
Dates: dry (1 cup chopped/178g)	2	11
Dates: dry (10 fruits/83g)	0	5
Elderberry: raw (½ cup/100g)	1	5
Feijoa: raw (1 fruit/50g)	0	1

	RiskPoints ✗	LifePoints ✔
Fig: canned in syrup, solids and liquid (3 fruits/85g)	0	1
Fig: dried, stewed (½ cup/130g)	1	5
Fig: dried, uncooked (5 fruits/90g)	2	7
Fig: raw (1 fruit/50g)	0	1
Fruit cocktail: (peach, pineapple, pear, grape and cherry) canned, in juice (½ cup/124g)	0	1
Fruit, mixed: (peach, cherry, raspberry, grape and boysenberry) frozen (½ cup thawed/125g)	0	0
Fruit, mixed: (peach, pear and pineapple) canned, in syrup (½ cup/128g)	0	2
Fruit, mixed: (prune, apricot and pear) dried (1 serving/100g)	1	6
Fruit salad: home-made (½ cup/128g)	0	3
Fruit salad: (peach, pear, apricot, pineapple and cherry) canned, in juice (½ cup/124g)	0	1
Fruit salad: tropical (pineapple, papaya, banana and guava) canned, in syrup (½ cup/128g)	0	2
Gooseberry: canned, in syrup (½ cup/126g)	0	2
Gooseberry: raw (1 cup/150g)	2	4
Gooseberry: stewed (½ cup/126g)	0	2
Granadilla: see 'Passion fruit'		
Grapefruit: juice, canned (1 cup/247g)	0	4
Grapefruit: juice, pink, raw (1 cup/247g)	0	5

	RiskPoints ✗	LifePoints ✔
Grapefruit: raw, pink and red (1 cup sections with juice/230g)	0	4
Grapefruit: raw, pink and red (½ fruit/123g)	0	2
Grapefruit: sections, canned, in juice (½ cup sections/124g)	0	2
Grape: canned, in syrup, Thompson seedless (½ cup/128g)	0	2
Grape: juice, canned or bottled (1 cup/253g)	0	3
Grape: European type, raw (10 fruits/50g)	0	1
Greengage: raw (1 cup slices/165g)	0	3
Greengage: raw (1 fruit/45g)	0	1
Groundcherry: raw (½ cup/70g)	1	2
Guava: raw (1 fruit/90g)	0	3
Guava: sauce, cooked (½ cup/119g)	10	53
Jackfruit: raw (1 serving/100g)	0	3
Jambolan: see 'Java plum'		
Japonica: see 'Loquat'		
Java plum: raw (1 cup/135g)	0	1
Jujube: dried (1 serving/100g)	2	6
Jujube: raw (1 serving/100g)	0	2
Kiwi fruit: raw (1 fruit/76g)	0	2
Kumquat: raw (1 fruit/19g)	0	0
Lemon: juice, canned or bottled (1 cup/244g)	1	4
Lemon: juice, canned or bottled (1 tbsp/15g)	0	0
Lemon: juice, raw (1 cup/244g)	0	5

	RiskPoints ✗	LifePoints ✔
Lemon: juice, raw (1 tbsp/15g)	0	0
Lemon: peel, raw (1 tbsp/6g)	0	0
Lemon: raw, without peel (1 fruit/58g)	0	1
Lime: raw (1 fruit/67g)	0	1
Loganberry: frozen (1 cup unthawed/147g)	1	6
Longan: dried (1 serving/100g)	1	8
Longan: raw (1 serving/100g)	0	2
Loquat: raw (1 cup/190g)	0	2
Lychee: canned, in syrup (½ cup/130g)	0	1
Lychee: dried (1 serving/100g)	3	10
Lychee: raw (1 cup/190g)	2	4
Mammy-apple: raw (½ fruit/423g)	5	7
Mandarin: see 'Tangerine'		
Mango: juice, canned (1 cup/251g)	1	3
Mango: raw (1 fruit/207g)	1	7
Marmalade plum: see 'Sapote'		
Melon: balls, frozen (1 cup/173g)	1	7
Melon: cantaloupe, raw (1 cup cubed pieces/160g)	1	6
Melon: cantaloupe, raw (½ fruit/267g)	1	6
Melon: honeydew, raw (1 cup cubed pieces/170g)	0	3
Mixed fruit: dried (1 handful/60g)	0	3
Mixed peel: (1oz/28g)	0	0
Mulberry: raw (10 fruits/15g)	0	0
Natal plum: see 'Carissa'		
Nectarine: raw (1 fruit/136g)	1	2

	RiskPoints ✗	LifePoints ✔
Olive: canned (1 small/3g)	0	0
Olive: canned (10 small/32g)	4	0
Orange: juice, canned (1 cup/249g)	0	7
Orange: juice, fresh (1 cup/249g)	1	9
Orange: juice, made from concentrate (1 cup/249g)	1	9
Orange: peel, raw (1 tbsp/6g)	0	0
Orange: raw (1 fruit/131g)	0	6
Orange: raw, with peel (1 fruit/159g)	1	7
Papaya: juice, canned (1 cup/250g)	0	2
Papaya: raw (1 fruit/304g)	1	12
Passion fruit: juice (1 cup/247g)	1	7
Passion fruit: raw (1 fruit/18g)	0	0
Peach: juice, canned, with added vitamin C (1 cup/249g)	0	2
Peach: juice, canned, without added vitamin C (1 cup/249g)	0	2
Peach: canned, in juice (1 half/77g)	0	1
Peach: dehydrated (low-moisture) sulphured, stewed (½ cup/121g)	1	4
Peach: dehydrated (low-moisture) sulphured, uncooked (½ cup/58g)	1	5
Peach: dried sulphured, stewed (½ cup halves/135g)	0	3
Peach: dried, sulphured, uncooked (10 halves/130g)	2	11
Peach: frozen (1 cup slices thawed/250g)	0	6
Peach: raw (1 cup slices/170g)	0	3
Peach: raw (1 fruit/87g)	0	1

	RiskPoints ✗	LifePoints ✔
Pear: juice, canned, with added vitamin C (1 cup/250g)	0	2
Pear: juice, canned, without added vitamin C (1 cup/250g)	0	1
Pear: canned, in juice (½ fruit/77g)	0	0
Pear: Chinese, raw (1 fruit/122g)	0	1
Pear: dried, sulphured, stewed (½ cup halves/128g)	0	3
Pear: dried, sulphured, uncooked (½ cup halves/90g)	1	4
Pear: raw (1 cup slices/165g)	1	2
Pear: raw (1 fruit/166g)	1	2
Persimmon: raw (1 fruit/25g)	0	0
Pineapple: canned, in juice (1 slice/58g)	0	1
Pineapple: chunks, frozen (½ cup chunks/122g)	0	3
Pineapple: juice, canned, with added vitamin C (1 cup/250g)	0	8
Pineapple: juice, canned, without added vitamin C (1 cup/250g)	0	7
Pineapple: juice, made from frozen concentrate (1 cup/250g)	0	5
Pineapple: raw (1 cup diced pieces/155g)	1	4
Pineapple: raw (1 slice/84g)	0	2
Pitanga: raw (½ cup/90g)	0	0
Plantain: cooked (½ cup slices/77g)	0	3
Plantain: raw (1 fruit/179g)	1	9
Plum: canned, in juice (3 fruits/95g)	0	1

	RiskPoints ✗	LifePoints ✔
Plum: raw (1 cup slices/165g)	2	3
Plum: raw (1 fruit/66g)	1	1
Plum: stewed (3 fruits/133g)	0	2
Poha: *see* 'Groundcherry'		
Pomegranate: juice, fresh (1 cup/251g)	0	5
Pomegranate: raw (1 fruit/154g)	1	2
Prickly pear: raw (1 fruit/103g)	1	2
Prune: canned, in syrup (5 fruits/86g)	0	3
Prune: dehydrated (low-moisture), stewed (½ cup/140g)	0	4
Prune: dehydrated (low-moisture), uncooked (½ cup/66g)	1	7
Prune: dried, stewed (½ cup/106g)	0	4
Prune: dried, uncooked (10 fruits/84g)	1	6
Prune: juice, canned (1 cup/256g)	0	8
Pummelo: raw (1 cup sections/190g)	0	3
Quince: raw (1 fruit/92g)	0	1
Raisin: golden seedless (1 cup/145g)	1	9
Raisin: seeded (1 cup/145g)	1	9
Raspberry: canned, in syrup (½ cup/128g)	0	3
Raspberry: frozen (½ cup/125g)	0	4
Raspberry: raw (1 cup/123g)	1	6
Raspberry: stewed (½ cup/128g)	0	3

	RiskPoints ✗	LifePoints ✔
Rhubarb: frozen, cooked (½ cup/120g)	0	3
Rhubarb: raw (½ cup diced pieces/61g)	0	1
Rose-apple: raw (1 serving/100g)	0	1
Roselle: raw (1 cup/57g)	0	2
Sapodilla: raw (1 fruit/170g)	4	3
Sapote: raw (1 fruit/225g)	3	7
Sharon fruit: raw (1 fruit/56g)	0	1
Soursop: raw (½ fruit/312g)	2	9
Starfruit: see 'Carambola'		
Strawberry: canned, in syrup (½ cup/127g)	0	4
Strawberry: frozen (1 cup unthawed/149g)	0	4
Strawberry: raw (1 cup/149g)	1	5
Sugar-apple: raw (1 fruit/155g)	1	7
Surinam cherry: see 'Pitanga'		
Sweetsop: see 'Sugar-apple'		
Tamarind: raw (1 cup pulp/120g)	2	10
Tangerine: canned in juice (½ cup/124g)	0	3
Tangerine: juice, canned (1 cup/249g)	1	4
Tangerine: juice, raw (1 cup/247g)	1	4
Tangerine: raw (1 fruit/84g)	0	3
Watermelon: raw (1 cup diced pieces/160g)	1	3

Breakfast Cereals

The average weight of most servings of breakfast cereals is about 30g: first choose your cereal, then add either whole, semi-skimmed, skimmed or soya milk as below.	RiskPoints ✘	LifePoints ✔
All Bran, Kellogg's: (standard serving 30g)	2	14
Banana Bubbles, Kellogg's: (standard serving 30g)	0	14
Bran Buds, Kellogg's: (standard serving 30g)	2	14
Bran Flakes, Kellogg's: (standard serving 30g)	1	17
Coco Pops, Kellogg's: (standard serving 30g)	1	14
Common Sense Oat Bran Flakes, Kellogg's: (standard serving 30g)	3	16
Common Sense Oat Bran Flakes, with Raisins and Apple, Kellogg's: (standard serving 30g)	3	12
Corn Flakes, Kellogg's: (standard serving 30g)	0	17
Corn Pops, Kellogg's: (standard serving 30g)	1	14
Country Store, Kellogg's: (standard serving 30g)	3	6
Crunchy Nut Corn Flakes, Kellogg's: (standard serving 30g)	2	14
Frosted Wheats, Kellogg's: (standard serving 30g)	1	12
Frosties, Kellogg's: (standard serving 30g)	0	14
Fruit 'n' Fibre, Kellogg's: (standard serving 30g)	6	12

	RiskPoints ✗	LifePoints ✔
Golden Crisp, Kellogg's: (standard serving 30g)	5	11
GrapeNuts: (standard serving 30g) ☺ *DietMentor*: This cereal is the basis for New Pastry, our high-LifePoints recipe in *LifePoints Cookbook*	0	25
Honey Nut Loops, Kellogg's: (standard serving 30g)	2	15
Muesli, swiss style: (standard 3oz serving 90g)	13	30
Multi-Grain Start, Kellogg's: (standard serving 30g)	1	18
Nut Feast, Kellogg's: (standard serving 30g)	6	12
Raisin Splitz, Kellogg's: (standard serving 30g)	1	12
Rice Krispies, Kellogg's: (standard serving 30g)	0	17
Ricicles, Kellogg's: (standard serving 30g)	0	14
Special K, Kellogg's: (standard serving 30g)	1	31
Sultana Bran, Kellogg's: (standard serving 30g)	1	13
Sustain, Kellogg's: (standard serving 30g)	2	14
Milk, cow's: Asda Light (virtually fat free) (¾ cup/183g)	0	9
Milk, cow's: semi-skimmed (¾ cup/183g)	13	10
Milk, cow's: skimmed (¾ cup/183g)	1	9
Milk, cow's: whole (¾ cup/183g)	32	9
Milk, goat's: (¾ cup/183g)	36	7
Milk, soya: (¾ cup/183g)	8	5

Cooked Breakfast Foods

	RiskPoints ✗	LifePoints ✔
For egg dishes, such as omelettes, hard boiled eggs, pancakes, etc. see Eggs in the Meat, Fish and Dairy group.		
Cream of rice: cooked with water (1 cup/244g)	0	2
Cream of wheat: instant, made with water (1 cup/241g)	1	11
Muffins: blueberry (commercial) (1 muffin/57g)	9	4
Muffins: corn (commercial) (1 muffin/57g)	11	6
Muffin: oat bran (1 muffin/57g)	10	6
Muffin: plain, prepared from recipe made with low-fat (2%) milk (1 muffin/57g)	16	6
Muffin: plain, prepared from recipe made with whole milk (1 muffin/57g)	17	6
Muffin: wheat bran, prepared from recipe made with whole milk (1 muffin/57g)	18	10
Porridge: made with semi-skimmed milk (¾ cup/210g)	19	5
Porridge: made with skimmed milk (¾ cup/210g)	5	14
Porridge: made with soya milk (¾ cup/207g)	12	10
Porridge: made with whole milk (¾ cup/210g)	33	14
Porridge oats: instant, made with water (1 pkt prepared/177g)	4	27
Waffles: plain, prepared from recipe (1 waffle/75g)	26	9
Waffles: plain, toasted (1 waffle/33g)	6	9

	RiskPoints ✗	LifePoints ✔
Waffles: potato, cooked from frozen (1 waffle/75g)	15	11

Breads

There is an infinite number of breads and bread products in the world, most of which are extremely delicious and very healthy, too. Here we've gathered comprehensive information on many of the most common kinds.	RiskPoints ✗	LifePoints ✔
Bagel: onion, poppy or sesame, toasted (1 bagel/66g)	2	4
Basic sandwich: 2 slices of wholewheat bread and margarine, add your own filling! (55g)	10	7
Bread: banana, made with margarine (1 slice/60g)	15	4
Bread: banana, made with vegetable shortening (1 slice/60g)	17	3
Bread: cornbread, made with low-fat milk (1 piece/60g)	10	7
Bread: cornbread, prepared from dry mix (1 piece/60g)	15	5
Bread: French (1 medium slice/25g)	1	3
Bread: granary (1 slice/33g)	1	5
Bread: Hovis granary (1 slice/33g)	1	5
Bread: Irish soda, prepared from recipe (1 slice/60g)	7	5
Bread: mixed-grain (1 slice/26g)	2	4
Bread: mixed-grain, toasted (1 slice/24g)	2	3
Bread: oat bran (1 slice/30g)	3	4

	RiskPoints ✗	LifePoints ✔
Bread: oat bran, toasted (1 slice/27g)	3	3
Bread: oatmeal (1 slice/27g)	2	3
Bread: oatmeal, toasted (1 slice/25g)	3	2
Bread: pumpernickel (1 slice/32g)	2	4
Bread: pumpernickel, toasted (1 slice/29g)	2	3
Bread: raisin (1 slice/26g)	2	3
Bread: raisin, toasted (1 slice/24g)	2	2
Bread: rye (1 slice/32g)	2	4
Bread: rye, toasted (1 slice/29g)	2	3
Bread: wheat germ, average (1 slice/30g)	1	4
Bread: wheat germ, toasted (1 slice/25g)	2	3
Bread: white (commercial) (1 slice/25g)	2	3
Bread: white (commercial) toasted (1 slice/23g)	2	3
Bread: wholewheat (commercial) (1 slice/25g)	2	3
Bread: wholewheat (commercial), toasted (1 slice/25g)	3	3
Breadcrumbs: dry, grated, plain (1 oz/28g)	3	6
Breadsticks: (1 average/15g)	6	0
Chapati: (1 medium made without fat/35g)	0	2
Croissant: apple (1 medium/57g)	18	4
Croissant: cheese (1 medium/57g)	41	8
Croissant: chocolate (1 medium/72g)	86	8

	RiskPoints ✗	LifePoints ✔
Croissant: plain (1 medium/57g)	28	6
☺ *DietMentor*: Would a toasted crumpet do? Try one spread with yeast extract or Bean Pâté for a high-LifePoints treat.		
Croissant: with egg and cheese (1 medium/127g)	105	16
Croissant: with egg, cheese and bacon (1 medium/129g)	115	17
Croissant: with egg, cheese and ham (1 medium/152g)	131	21
Croissant: with egg, cheese and sausage (1 medium/160g)	136	24
Crumpet: fresh (1 average/60g)	1	3
Crumpet: toasted (1 average/60g)	1	3
Currant bun: (1 average/66g)	12	7
French toast: frozen, ready to heat (1 piece/59g)	8	11
French toast: with butter (2 slices/135g)	58	16
Hot cross bun: (1 average/66g)	11	5
Maltbread: (1 slice/30g)	1	3
Milk bread: (1 slice/30g)	6	3
Naan bread: (1 medium/90g)	28	7
Papadum: fried (1 average/15g)	6	2
Papadum: raw (1 average/10g)	0	2
Paratha: (1 average/90g)	32	8
Pitta: white (1 average/60g)	1	4
☺ *DietMentor*: a versatile bread that is delicious stuffed with salads, Bean Pâté or even asparagus tips with a low-fat dressing.		

	RiskPoints ✗	LifePoints ✔
Pitta: wholewheat (1 average/64g)	4	8
Pizza: cheese and tomato (1 slice/70g)	28	6
Pizza: cheese and tomato, retail, frozen (1 slice/70g)	22	5
Pizza: cheese and tomato, wholemeal (1 slice/70g) ☺ DietMentor: In a restaurant, ask for the Marinara without the anchovies. A sprinkling of fresh basil makes this superb.	28	8
Puri: Punjabi (1 average/20g)	17	2
Roll: dinner, plain (commercial) (1 average/66g)	12	9
Roll: hamburger or hotdog, plain (1 roll/43g)	5	5
Scone: cheese (1 average/80g)	35	7
Scone: fruit (1 average/80g)	19	6
Scone: plain (1 average/80g)	29	6
Scone: potato (1 average/80g)	28	4
Scone: wholemeal (1 average/80g)	28	9
Scone: wholemeal, fruit (1 average/80g)	25	8
Stuffing: bread, dry mix, prepared (1 oz/28g)	6	1
Teacake: fresh (1 average/60g)	11	5
Teacake: toasted (1 average/55g)	11	5
Toast: wholewheat, with butter (1 slice/30g)	20	4
Toast: wholewheat, with margarine (1 slice/30g)	13	4
Toast: wholewheat, with olive oil (1 slice/30g)	15	3

	RiskPoints ✗	LifePoints ✔
Tortilla: made with wheat flour (1 medium/35g)	0	2

Crackers

	RiskPoints ✗	LifePoints ✔
Cracker: brown wheat (3 thin square crackers/6g)	3	0
Cracker: brown wheat, sandwich, with cheese filling (1 sandwich cracker/7g)	4	1
Cracker: brown, wholewheat (3 square crackers/12g)	5	1
Cracker: cocktail, cheese (10 × 1 in square crackers/10g)	7	2
Cracker: snack-type (3 round crackers/9g)	5	1
Cracker: snack-type, sandwich, with cheese filling (1 sandwich cracker/7g)	3	1
Cracker: soup cracker (3 crackers/9g)	2	1
Cracker: cream cracker (1 cracker/7g)	2	0
Cracker: crispbread, rye (1 piece/6g)	0	0
Cracker: crispbread, rye (1 wafer/10g)	0	1
Cracker: matzo (1 cracker/4g)	0	0
Cracker: matzo, wholewheat (1 large/28g)	1	5
Cracker: matzo, with egg (1 large/28g)	1	5
Cracker: matzo, with egg and onion (1 large/28g)	2	4
Cracker: Melba toast, rye (includes pumpernickel) (1 toast/5g)	0	0

	RiskPoints ✘	LifePoints ✔
Cracker: oatcake, home-made (1 cake/15g)	6	1
Cracker: oatcake, retail (1 cake/15g)	6	1
Cracker: pretzel (10 twists/60g)	5	8
Cracker: rice cake, with brown rice and buckwheat (2 cakes/18g)	1	2
☺ DietMentor: Use these cakes as a platform for creative, high-LifePoints snacks and lunches.		
Cracker: rice cake, with brown rice and corn (2 cakes/18g)	1	1
Cracker: rice cake, with brown rice and sesame seed (2 cakes/18g)	1	2
Cracker: rice cake, with brown rice, multigrain (2 cakes/18g)	1	2
Cracker: rice cakes, with brown rice, plain (2 cakes/18g)	1	2
Cracker: rice cake, with brown rice and rye (2 cakes/18g)	1	1
Cracker: water biscuit (3 biscuits/15g)	4	1
Cracker: zwiebäck (1 piece/7g)	2	0

Grains & Flours

	RiskPoints ✘	LifePoints ✔
Amaranth: (½ cup/98g)	15	17
Arrowroot: flour (1 tbsp/10g)	0	0
Arrowroot: flour (½ cup/64g)	0	1
Barley: pearled, cooked (½ cup/79g)	0	4
Buckwheat: flour, whole-groat (½ cup/60g)	4	12
Buckwheat: groats, roasted, cooked (½ cup/99g)	1	3

	RiskPoints ✗	LifePoints ✓
Bulghur: cooked (½ cup/91g) ☺ *DietMentor*: Quicker than brown rice and with a lovely nutty flavour. Much used in Middle Eastern cookery.	0	4
Burrito: with beans (2 burritos/217g)	51	28
Burrito: with beans and cheese (2 burritos/186g)	51	23
Burrito: with beans and chilli peppers (2 burritos/204g)	57	29
Burrito: with beans and meat (2 burritos/231g)	62	33
Burrito: with beans, cheese and beef (2 burritos/203g)	53	24
Burrito: with beans, cheese and chilli peppers (2 burritos/336g)	83	48
Burrito: with beef (2 burritos/220g)	78	32
Burrito: with beef and chilli peppers (2 burritos/201g)	59	27
Burrito: with beef, cheese and chilli peppers (2 burritos/304g)	77	46
Burrito: with fruit (apple or cherry) 1 small burrito/74g)	34	7
Chimichanga: with beef (1 chimichanga/174g)	63	28
Chimichanga: with beef and cheese (1 chimichanga/183g)	83	27
Chimichanga: with beef and red chilli peppers (1 chimichanga/190g)	62	23
Chimichanga: with beef, cheese and red chilli peppers (1 chimichanga/180g)	62	25

	RiskPoints ✗	LifePoints ✔
Coo-coo: cornmeal, with okra (1 serving/210g)	11	3
Corn: cooked (½ cup/70g)	1	2
Corn: flour, wholegrain, yellow (½ cup/58g)	5	7
Corn: fritters, fried in vegetable oil (1 fritter/55g)	21	3
Corn: pudding (⅔ cup/167g)	31	13
Cornmeal: wholegrain, yellow (½ cup/61g)	5	8
Cornstarch: (⅓ cup/43g)	0	0
Couscous: cooked (½ cup/90g) ☺ DietMentor: Buy the quick to prepare type and you can eat it within ten minutes. Use in salads, soups and under a sauce or stew.	0	3
Couscous: made with chickpeas and mixed vegetables (1 serving/179g)	16	10
Dumplings: (2 average/60g)	29	2
Enchilada: with cheese (1 enchilada/163g)	79	17
Enchilada: with cheese and beef (1 enchilada/192g)	67	24
Enchirito: with cheese, beef and beans (1 enchirito/193g)	59	30
French toast: prepared from recipe, made with whole milk (1 slice/65g)	18	6
Frijoles: with cheese (1 serving/167g)	30	19
Hominy: canned, white (½ cup/80g)	1	1
Millet: cooked (½ cup/120g)	3	6

	RiskPoints ✗	LifePoints ✔
Nacho: with cheese (6–8 nachos/113g)	58	15
Nacho: with cheese and jalapeño peppers (6–8 nachos/204g)	105	24
Nacho: with cheese, beans, ground beef and peppers (6–8 nachos/255g)	93	26
Nacho: with cinnamon and sugar (6–8 nachos/109g)	136	17
Oat: bran, cooked (½ cup/110g)	2	3
Oat: bran, raw (½ cup/47g)	8	11
Oat: raw (½ cup/78g)	13	14
Pastry: filo (1 sheet pastry/19g)	2	2
Pastry: puff, frozen, ready to bake, baked (1 oz/28g) ☺ DietMentor: See our New Pastry in LifePoints Cookbook (5 RiskPoints, 28 LifePoints)	27	2
Quinoa: (½ cup/85g)	12	16
Ravioli: with spinach and cheese filling (1 serving/240g)	41	23
Rice: bran, crude (½ cup/42g)	21	32
Rice: brown, long-grain cooked (½ cup/98g)	2	3
Rice: brown, medium-grain cooked (½ cup/98g)	2	3
Rice: flour, brown (½ cup/79g)	5	12
Rice: flour, white (½ cup/79g)	2	5
Rice: pilau, plain (1 serving/195g)	36	6
Rice: rissole, fried in sunflower oil (2 rissoles/120g)	26	8
Rice: rissole, fried in vegetable oil (2 rissoles/120g)	26	8

	RiskPoints ✗	LifePoints ✔
Rice: salad (brown rice, vegetables, nuts and raisins) (1 serving/200g)	37	9
Rice: salad (white rice, vegetables, nuts and raisins (1 serving/200g)	37	9
Rice: white, glutinous, cooked (½ cup/120g)	0	1
Rice: white, long-grain, regular, cooked (½ cup/79g)	0	3
Rice: white, medium-grain, cooked (½ cup/93g)	0	3
Rice: white, short-grain, cooked (½ cup/93g)	0	3
Rice: brown, with blackeye beans (West Indian) (1 serving/240g)	27	20
Rice: white, with blackeye beans (West Indian) (1 serving/240g)	27	20
Rice: brown, with pigeon peas, (West Indian) (1 serving/240g)	25	14
Rice: white, with pigeon peas, (West Indian) (1 serving/240g)	25	12
Rice: brown, with red kidney beans, (West Indian) (1 serving/240g)	25	15
Rice: white, with red kidney beans, (West Indian) (1 serving/240g)	27	15
Rice: white, with spinach pilaf (1 serving/180g)	11	19
Rice: brown, with split peas (West Indian) (1 serving/240g)	28	14
Rice: white, with split peas (West Indian) (1 serving/240g)	28	14
Rice: white, with tomato pilaf (1 serving/180g)	14	6

	RiskPoints ✗	LifePoints ✔
Risotto: alla milanese, with meat (1 serving/225g)	35	16
☺ *DietMentor*: Risotto is made with lots and lots of oil. Try our suggestions for a wild rice risotto instead, see page 218.		
Risotto: alla piemontese, vegetarian, with Parmesan cheese (1 serving/150g)	36	6
Risotto: vegetable, with brown rice (1 serving/180g)	28	11
Risotto: vegetable, with white rice (1 serving/180g)	29	11
Rye: flour, dark (½ cup/64g)	4	15
Rye: flour, light (½ cup/51g)	1	5
Rye: flour, medium (½ cup/51g)	2	6
Semolina: enriched (½ cup/84g)	2	18
Taco: (1 small taco/171g)	85	21
Taco: salad (1 serving/198g)	51	16
Taco: salad, with chilli con carne (1 serving/261g)	45	22
Taco: shell, baked (1 medium/13g)	7	1
Toaster: pastry fruit (includes apple, blueberry, cherry, strawberry) (1 pastry/52g)	13	8
Toaster: pastry, brown sugar and cinnamon (1 pastry/50g)	17	9
Tortilla: ready to bake or fry, corn (1 medium/25g)	1	2
Tortilla: ready to bake or fry, flour (1 medium/35g)	6	4
Tostada: with beans and cheese (1 tostada/144g)	40	16

	RiskPoints ✗	LifePoints ✔
Tostada: with beans, beef and cheese (1 tostada/225g)	86	23
Tostada: with beef and cheese (1 tostada/163g)	77	21
Tostada: with guacamole (1 tostada/130g)	36	12
Triticale: flour, wholegrain (½ cup/65g)	2	12
Wheat: bran, crude (½ cup/30g)	3	13
Wheat: bran, crude (2 tbsp/7g)	0	3
Wheat: flour, white, all-purpose, enriched bleached (½ cup/62g)	1	11
Wheat: flour, white, all-purpose, self-raising enriched (½ cup/62g)	1	12
Wheat: flour, white, bread, enriched (½ cup/69g)	2	13
Wheat: flour, white, cake, enriched (½ cup/54g)	1	10
Wheat: flour, wholegrain (½ cup/60g)	2	11
Wheat: flour, wholemeal, Doves Farm strong, organic (½ cup/58g)	2	11
Wheat: germ, crude (½ cup/58g)	14	32
Wheat: germ, crude (2 tbsp/14g)	3	8
Wheat: sprouted (½ cup/54g)	1	5
Wild rice: cooked (½ cup/82g) ☺ DietMentor: Eat lots of this! It can be expensive, so mix it with equal parts of brown rice, millet and/or barley for a nutty risotto.	0	4
Wonton: wrappers (includes egg roll wrappers) (1 wrapper/8g)	0	1
Yorkshire pudding: 1 individual pudding/30g)	10	1

Pasta

	RiskPoints ✗	LifePoints ✔
Cannelloni: with cheesy vegetable filling (3 shells/300g)	76	10
Cannelloni: with meat filling (3 shells/300g)	42	24
Cannelloni: with spinach and ricotta filling (3 shells/300g)	56	12
Lasagne: made with beef mince and Parmesan (1 serving/300g)	75	34
Lasagne: made with TVP mince and Parmesan (1 serving/300g) ☺ *DietMentor*: Simply substitute the TVP mince for the beef in your favourite recipe.	25	44
Macaroni: cheese, canned (1 serving/205g)	35	11
Macaroni: cheese, home-made from traditional recipe, with milk, margarine and cheese (1 serving/200g) ☺ *DietMentor*: Try our Macaroni in Mustard Sauce instead, see *LifePoints Cookbook*.	84	14
Macaroni: plain, cooked (1 cup/115g)	0	7
Macaroni: vegetable, cooked (1 cup/134g)	0	5
Macaroni: wholewheat, cooked (1 cup/140g)	1	6
Noodles: Chinese, chow mein (1 cup/45g)	34	7
Noodles: egg, cooked (1 cup/160g)	5	9
Noodles: egg, spinach, cooked (1 cup/160g)	6	12

	RiskPoints ✗	LifePoints ✔
Noodles: Japanese soba, cooked (1 cup/114g)	0	3
Noodles: Japanese somen, cooked (1 cup/176g)	0	2
Pasta: fresh-refrigerated, plain, cooked (1 cup/140g)	3	8
Pasta: fresh-refrigerated, spinach, cooked (1 cup/140g)	3	9
Pasta: home-made, made with egg, cooked (1 cup/140g)	6	8
Pasta: home-made, made without egg, cooked (1 cup/140g)	3	7
Pasta: salad (pasta, vegetables and mayonnaise (1 serving/180g)	33	7
Pasta: salad (wholemeal pasta, vegetables and mayonnaise) (1 serving/180g)	33	10
Pasta: with bean soup (1 cup/253g)	12	10
Pasticcio: (Greek: macaroni, lentils and vegetables with white sauce) (1 serving/180g)	48	12
Spaghetti: Bolognese (1 serving/410g) ☺ DietMentor: Substitute TVP mince for the beef in your favourite Bolognese sauce to turn it into a high-LifePoints meal.	57	32
Spaghetti: canned, Asda Healthy Choice (lower in sugar and salt) (½ can/205g)	0	10
Spaghetti: cooked (1 cup/140g)	2	7
Spaghetti: in four cheeses sauce (Gruyère, fontina, Parmesan and mozzarella (1 serving/449g)	317	42

	RiskPoints ✗	LifePoints ✔
Spaghetti: wholewheat, cooked (1 cup/140g)	1	6
Spaghetti: with Italian sauce (tomatoes, mushrooms, ham, olive oil) (1 serving/382g)	49	18
Spaghetti: with pesto sauce (1 cup/150g)	25	9
Spaghetti: with simple tomato sauce (made from tomatoes, onion, garlic, olive oil and green pepper) (1 serving/300g)	26	11
Tagliatelle: with vegetables, retail (1 serving/300g)	22	5

General

	RiskPoints ✗	LifePoints ✔
Ackee: canned, drained (1 average serving/115g)	43	6
Agar: dried (1 tsp/3g) ☺ DietMentor: Use instead of gelatine to make jellies and blancmanges.	0	0
Amaranth: boiled, drained (½ cup/66g)	0	6
Amaranth: leaves, boiled in unsalted water (1 cup/136g)	1	13
Arrowhead: boiled in unsalted water (1 medium corm/12g)	0	0
Artichoke: globe, boiled (1 medium/128g) ☺ DietMentor: Traditionally served with garlic butter, try a low-fat dressing instead to keep the RiskPoints low.	0	2
Artichoke: Jerusalem, boiled (4 small pieces/100g)	0	1
Asparagus: boiled (4 large spears/100g) ☺ DietMentor: We steam these, with the thick stalks in the boiling water. A low-fat dressing or vegetable purée is a perfect accompaniment.	1	5
Asparagus: raw (4 large spears/135g)	2	13

	RiskPoints ✗	LifePoints ✔
Asparagus: soup, cream of, canned, made with equal volume of milk (1 cup/248g)	24	10
Asparagus: soup, cream of, canned, made with equal volume of water (1 cup/244g)	10	4
Asparagus: soup, cream of, dehydrated, made with water (1 cup/251g)	4	2
Asparagus: tips, canned, drained (½ cup/121g)	1	10
Aubergine: curry (1 average serving/115g)	29	3
Aubergine: fried in corn oil (1 average serving/115g) ☺ DietMentor: Aubergine is a sponge for oils and fats; be careful!	91	1
Aubergine: pakora/bhaji, fried in vegetable oil (1 pakora/25g)	14	2
Aubergine: stuffed with lentils and vegetables (1 average serving/115g)	13	3
Aubergine: stuffed with rice (1 average serving/115g)	6	3
Aubergine: stuffed with vegetables, cheese topping (1 average serving/115g)	31	8
Aubergine: with pea, potato and cauliflower bhaji (1 average serving/115g)	7	7
Aubergine: with potato bhaji (1 average serving/115g)	25	5
Balsam-pear: (bitter melon) leafy tips, boiled (½ cup/29g)	0	4

	RiskPoints ✗	LifePoints ✓
Balsam-pear: pods, boiled (½ cup/62g)	0	3
Bamboo: shoots, canned (½ can/131g)	0	3
Bamboo: shoots, stir-fried (1 cup slices/125g)	13	2
Bean sprouts: mung, boiled (½ cup/62g)	0	3
Bean sprouts: mung, canned, drained (½ cup/62g)	0	1
Bean sprouts: mung, raw (½ cup/52g) ☺ DietMentor: Not just a garnish – stuff these into pitta for a light, low-RiskPoints snack.	0	3
Bean sprouts: mung, stir-fried in blended oil (½ cup/62g)	9	2
Beet: greens, boiled (1 cup/144g) ☺ DietMentor: Mix these greens with others such as dandelion, chicory and kale to give a deep, textured flavour. Sprinkle with black pepper and a little lemon juice just before serving.	0	12
Beetroot: boiled (2 beets/100g)	0	7
Beetroot: canned (½ cup/123g)	0	4
Beetroot: harvard, in butter, sugar and vinegar sauce (½ cup slices/122g)	9	5
Beetroot: pickled (½ cup slices/120g)	0	2
Beetroot: raw (½ cup slices/68g)	0	6
Beetroot: salad (1 average serving/115g)	19	7

	RiskPoints ✗	LifePoints ✔
Breadfruit: boiled (1 average serving/115g)	1	2
Breadfruit: canned (1 average serving/115g)	0	3
Broccoli: boiled (1 spear/180g)	3	12
Broccoli: flan (1 average serving/115g)	50	11
Broccoli: flan, wholemeal (1 average serving/115g)	50	13
Broccoli: frozen, boiled (1 average serving/115g)	2	8
Broccoli: green, raw, flower clusters (½ cup chopped/44g) ☺ *DietMentor*: Arrange these round a bowl of low-fat dip or salsa for an attractive, high-LifePoints snack.	0	4
Broccoli: green, raw, leaves (½ cup chopped/44g)	0	5
Broccoli: green, raw, whole (1 spear/150g)	3	8
Broccoli: in cheese sauce, made with semi-skimmed milk (1 average serving/115g)	32	10
Broccoli: in cheese sauce, made with skimmed milk (1 average serving/115g)	29	10
Broccoli: in cheese sauce, made with whole milk (1 average serving/115g)	37	10
Broccoli: purple sprouting, boiled (1 spear/110g)	1	13
Broccoli: purple sprouting, raw (1 spear/90g)	2	15

	RiskPoints ✗	LifePoints ✔
Brussels sprouts: boiled (5 sprouts/100g)	3	9
Brussels sprouts: canned (5 sprouts/100g)	2	1
Brussels sprouts: frozen, boiled (5 sprouts/100g)	3	7
Brussels sprouts: raw (5 sprouts/55g) ☺ DietMentor: Yes! You can eat them raw - they are delicious finely chopped into a salad.	1	7
Bubble and squeak: fried in lard (1 average serving/15g)	31	4
Bubble and squeak: fried in sunflower oil (1 average serving/115g)	26	4
Bubble and squeak: fried in vegetable oil (1 average serving/115g)	26	4
Burdock: root, boiled (1 cup/125g)	0	5
Cabbage: bhaji (1 average serving/115g)	14	8
Cabbage: Chinese (pak-choi), boiled (1 cup shredded/170g)	0	10
Cabbage: Chinese (pak-choi), raw (1 cup shredded/70g)	0	5
Cabbage: Chinese (pe-tsai), boiled (1 cup shredded/119g)	0	6
Cabbage: Chinese (pe-tsai) raw (1 cup shredded/76g)	0	6
Cabbage: curry (1 average serving/115g)	14	5
Cabbage: red, boiled (1 cup/145g)	1	5

	RiskPoints ✗	LifePoints ✔
Cabbage: red, cooked with apple (1 cup/145g)	10	4
Cabbage: red, raw (1 cup/70g)	0	3
Cabbage: Savoy, boiled (1 cup/145g)	1	7
Cabbage: Savoy, raw (1 cup/70g)	0	9
Cabbage: summer, boiled (1 cup/145g)	1	4
Cabbage: summer, raw (1 cup/70g)	0	3
Cabbage: white, boiled (1 cup/145g)	1	5
Cabbage: white, raw (1 cup/70g)	0	3
Cabbage: with pea bhaji, with butter ghee (1 average serving/115g)	81	9
Cabbage: with pea bhaji, with vegetable oil (1 average serving/115g)	42	8
Cabbage: with potato bhaji, with butter (1 average serving/115g)	31	8
Cabbage: with potato bhaji, with vegetable oil (1 average serving/115g)	20	7
Cabbage: with spinach bhaji (1 average serving/115g)	49	11
Cailalo: and okra (West Indian) (1 average serving/115g)	25	7
Cailalo: and cho cho (West Indian) (1 average serving/115g)	25	5
Cardoon: boiled (1 average serving/115g)	0	3

	RiskPoints ✗	LifePoints ✔
Carrot: baby, raw (1 average serving/115g)	1	5
Carrot: canned (½ cup slices/123g)	0	3
Carrot: frozen, boiled (½ cup slices/73g)	0	3
Carrot: juice (1 cup/246g) ☺ *DietMentor*: Add a pinch of freshly grated ginger for a really zingy drink.	0	14
Carrot: old, boiled (½ cup slices/78g)	0	4
Carrot: old, raw (1 medium carrot/72g)	0	4
Carrot: old, raw (½ cup shredded/55g)	0	3
Carrot: with nut salad, with mayonnaise, retail (1 average serving/115g)	71	9
Carrot: with orange soup (1 cup/240g)	3	5
Carrot: with potato and pea bhaji, with butter (1 average serving/115g)	36	8
Carrot: with potato and pea bhaji, with vegetable oil (1 average serving/115g)	23	7
Carrot: young, boiled (½ cup slices/78g)	0	3
Carrot: young, raw (1 medium carrot/72g)	0	4
Carrot: young, raw (½ cup shredded/55g)	0	3
Cassava: baked (1 average serving/115g)	0	3

	RiskPoints ✘	LifePoints ✔
Cassava: boiled (1 average serving/115g)	0	2
Cassava: chips (1 average serving/115g)	1	3
Cassava: gari (1 average serving/115g)	1	5
Cassava: steamed (1 average serving/115g)	0	3
Cauliflower: bhaji (1 average serving/115g)	58	8
Cauliflower: boiled (½ cup pieces/62g)	1	3
Cauliflower (3 florets/54g)	1	3
Cauliflower: cheese flan (1 average serving/115g)	43	6
Cauliflower: cheese flan, wholemeal (1 average serving/115g)	43	8
Cauliflower: cheese, made with semi-skimmed milk (1 average serving/115g)	25	9
Cauliflower: cheese, made with skimmed milk (1 average serving/115g) ☺ *DietMentor*: Or try our version of this old classic: Cauliflower in Mustard Sauce in *LifePoints Cookbook*	24	9
Cauliflower: cheese, made with whole milk (1 average serving/115g)	29	9
Cauliflower: curry, gobi aloo sag, retail (1 average serving/115g)	19	5
Cauliflower: frozen, boiled (½ cup pieces/90g)	1	3

	RiskPoints ✗	LifePoints ✔
Cauliflower: in white sauce, made with semi-skimmed milk (1 average serving/115g)	9	6
Cauliflower: in white sauce, made with skimmed milk (1 average serving/115g)	7	6
Cauliflower: in white sauce, made with whole milk (1 average serving/115g)	13	6
Cauliflower: pakora/bhaji, fried in vegetable oil (1 pakora/25g)	15	3
Cauliflower: potato and pea bhaji, with butter (1 average serving/115g)	61	8
Cauliflower: potato and pea bhaji, with vegetable oil (1 average serving/115g)	39	7
Cauliflower: raw (½ cup pieces/50g)	1	4
Cauliflower: raw (3 florets/56g)	1	4
Cauliflower: soup, dehydrated, made with water (1 cup/256g)	4	3
Cauliflower: with onions and chilli pepper (1 average serving/115g)	9	6
Cauliflower: with potato bhaji (1 average serving/115g)	20	9
Cauliflower: with potato curry (1 average serving/115g)	6	7
Cauliflower: with vegetable pakora/bhaji (1 pakora/25g)	10	2
Celeriac: boiled (½ cup/78g)	0	3
Celeriac: raw (½ cup/78g)	0	5
Celery: boiled (½ cup diced/75g)	0	1
Celery: raw (1 stalk/40g)	0	1
Celery: raw (½ cup diced/60g)	0	1

	RiskPoints ✗	LifePoints ✓
Celery: soup, cream of, canned, made with equal volume of milk (1 cup/248g)	29	8
Celery: soup, cream of, canned, made with equal volume of water (1 cup/244g)	13	3
Celery: soup, cream of, dehydrated, made with water (1 cup/254g)	4	2
Chard: Swiss, boiled (½ cup chopped/88g)	0	8
Chard: Swiss, raw (1 leaf/48g)	0	6
Chicory: greens, raw (½ cup chopped/90g)	0	10
Chicory: roots, raw (½ cup pieces/45g)	0	1
Chicory: witloof raw (½ cup/45g)	0	1
Chives: raw (1 tbsp chopped/3g)	0	0
Cho Cho: boiled in unsalted water (1 average serving/115g)	0	1
Cho Cho: fritters, fried in vegetable oil (1 fritter/55g)	17	3
Cho Cho: raw (½ cup/90g)	0	1
Coco: fritters, fried in vegetable oil (1 fritter/55g)	31	3
Cole: leaves, dried, boiled (½ cup/107g)	2	3
Coleslaw: (½ cup/60g)	16	2
Coleslaw: with mayonnaise, retail (½ cup/60g)	39	3
Coleslaw: with reduced-calorie dressing, retail (½ cup/60g)	6	2
Coleslaw: with vinaigrette, retail (½ cup/60g)	6	2

	RiskPoints ✗	LifePoints ✔
Collards: boiled (½ cup chopped/64g)	0	1
Collards: frozen, boiled (½ cup chopped/85g)	0	9
Collards: raw (½ cup chopped/18g)	0	0
Corn: on the cob, with butter (1 ear/146g) ☺ *DietMentor*: We know it's delicious, but try it with a tablespoon of low-fat French dressing instead of butter.	12	9
Corn: with red and green peppers, canned (½ cup/114g)	1	5
Corn salad: raw (½ cup/28g)	0	2
Courgette: boiled (½ cup mashed/120g) ☺ *DietMentor*: Stir some freshly ground pepper and finely chopped spring onions into this mash and spread on crisp toast for a luscious snack.	1	4
Courgette: boiled (½ cup slices/90g)	0	3
Courgette: fried in corn oil (½ cup slices/90g)	10	5
Courgette: raw (½ cup slices/65g)	0	3
Courgette: with potato curry (1 average serving/115g)	14	5
Courgette: with eggs (1 average serving/115g)	29	8
Cress: garden, raw (½ cup/25g)	0	3
Cucumber: raw (1 cucumber/301g)	0	5

	RiskPoints ✗	LifePoints ✔
Cucumber: raw (½ cup slices/52g)	0	0
Curly kale: boiled (½ cup chopped/65g)	1	7
Curly kale: raw (½ cup chopped/34g)	1	5
Dandelion: greens, boiled (½ cup chopped/52g)	0	4
Dandelion: greens, raw (½ cup chopped/28g) ☺ *DietMentor*: If your supermarket hasn't got any yet, try your local Greek or Asian grocer. These greens are a must.	0	3
Dosa: filling, vegetable (1 average serving/115g)	18	5
Drumstick leaves: boiled (1 average serving/115g)	2	22
Drumstick leaves: raw (½ cup chopped/67g)	2	24
Endive: raw (½ cup chopped/25g)	0	2
Fennel: Florence, boiled (1 bulb/234g)	1	7
Fennel: Florence, raw (1 bulb/234g) ☺ *DietMentor*: Grate this together with a large, sweet apple, add a tablespoon of plain low-fat yogurt, some finely chopped spring onions and dip to your heart's content.	1	9
Fennel: Florence, raw (1 cup sliced/87g)	0	3

233

	RiskPoints ✗	LifePoints ✔
Fenugreek: leaves, raw (½ cup chopped/28g)	0	3
Fu-Fu: West Indian dish made with sweet potato (1 average serving/115g)	1	5
Fu-Fu: West Indian dish made with yam (1 average serving/115g)	1	4
Garlic: purée (1 tbsp/15g)	12	0
Garlic: purée (½ cup/125g)	105	2
Garlic: raw (3 cloves/9g)	0	0
Gazpacho: canned (1 cup/244g)	5	5
Gazpacho: traditional recipe (1 cup/244g)	21	5
Gherkins: pickled (5 average/30g)	0	0
Ginger: root, raw (¼ cup slices/24g)	0	0
Gourd: kantola, canned (½ cup cubes/73g)	1	4
Gourd: karela, bhaji, with butter ghee (1 average serving/115g)	56	6
Gourd: karela, bhaji, with vegetable oil (1 average serving/115g)	30	6
Gourd: karela, canned (½ cup cubes/73g)	0	2
Gourd: karela, curry (1 average serving/115g)	28	5
Gourd: tinda, canned (½ cup cubed/73g)	0	1
Gourd: tinda with potato curry (1 average serving/115g)	11	2
Gourd: white-flowered (calabash) boiled (½ cup cubes/73g)	0	1
Guacamole: (½ cup/138g)	43	6

	RiskPoints ✗	LifePoints ✔
Horseradish: raw (1 heaped tbsp gratings/20g)	0	1
Irish moss: raw (1 cup/145g)	0	14
Kale: boiled (½ cup chopped/65g)	0	4
Kale: raw (½ cup chopped/34g)	0	3
Kale: Scotch, boiled (½ cup chopped/65g)	0	3
Kale: Scotch, raw (½ cup chopped/34g)	0	3
Kelp: raw (1 cup/145g)	2	16
Kohlrabi: boiled (1 average serving/115g)	0	5
Kohlrabi: raw (½ cup slices/68g) ☺ *DietMentor:* Grate or thinly slice this delicate root, drizzle with lemon juice and a pinch of pepper or nutmeg and serve. Yummy!	0	4
Kombu: dried, raw (1 strip/30g) ☺ *DietMentor:* Add one of these to every soup or stew you ever make for a LifePoints lift that also adds depth of flavour.	1	10
Lambsquarters: boiled (½ cup chopped/90g)	1	9
Lambsquarters: raw (½ cup/50g)	1	8
Laverbread: (1 average serving/115g)	10	8
Leek: and potato soup (1 cup/250g)	30	7
Leek: and potato soup, made with cream (1 cup/250g)	20	7

	RiskPoints ✗	LifePoints ✔
Leek: boiled (1 leek/124g)	2	5
☺ DietMentor: Steam one leek per person, leave to cool and then dress in low-fat French dressing for an exotic starter or snack.		
Leek: boiled (½ cup chopped/52g)	0	2
Leek: in cheese sauce, made with semi-skimmed milk (1 average serving/115g)	25	7
Leek: in cheese sauce, made with skimmed milk (1 average serving/115g)	23	7
Leek: in cheese sauce, made with whole milk (1 average serving/115g)	30	7
Leek: raw (1 leek/124g)	1	12
Leek: raw (½ cup chopped/52g)	0	5
Leek: soup, dehydrated, made with water (1 cup/254g)	7	2
Lettuce: average, raw (½ cup shredded/28g)	0	1
Lettuce: butterhead, raw (½ cup shredded/28g)	0	1
Lettuce: cos, raw (½ cup shredded/28g)	0	1
Lettuce: iceberg, raw (½ cup shredded/28g)	0	1
Lettuce: webbs, raw (½ cup shredded/28g)	0	1
Lotus: tubers, canned (10 slices/89g)	0	0
Lotus: tubers, raw (1 root 9 in. long/115g)	0	3
Marrow: boiled (½ cup cubes/58g)	0	1

	RiskPoints ✘	LifePoints ✔
Marrow: parwal, canned (½ cup cubes/58g)	0	2
Marrow: parwal, raw (½ cup cubes/58g)	0	2
Marrow: raw (½ cup cubes/58g)	0	1
Matoki: boiled (½ cup slices/77g)	0	4
Matoki: raw (½ cup slices/74g)	0	5
Mchicha: (West Indian: steamed spinach with onion and tomato) (1 average serving/115g)	13	17
Minestrone: soup, canned (1 cup/246g)	7	4
Minestrone: soup, canned, made with equal volume of water (1 cup/241g)	6	5
Minestrone: soup, home-made (1 cup/241g)	18	6
Minestrone: soup, canned, chunky, ready to serve (1 cup/240g)	11	9
Minestrone: soup, dehydrated, made with water (1 cup/254g)	6	4
Moussaka: vegetable, retail (1 average serving/115g)	14	5
Mushroom: bhaji (1 average serving/115g)	46	6
Mushroom: boiled (½ cup pieces/78g)	0	4
Mushroom: canned (½ cup pieces/78g)	0	3
Mushroom: Chinese, dried (4 mushrooms/15g)	0	4
Mushroom: common, raw (1 mushroom/18g)	0	1

	RiskPoints ✘	LifePoints ✔
Mushroom: common, raw (½ cup pieces/35g)	0	2
Mushroom: dopiaza, retail (1 average serving/115g)	16	4
Mushroom: fried in corn oil (1 average serving/115g)	46	8
Mushroom: garlic, sauté in butter (1 average serving/115g)	79	8
Mushroom: Jew's ear, tender, dried, soaked, raw (½ cup/12g)	0	0
Mushroom: Jew's ear, tough, dried, soaked, raw (½ cup/12g)	0	0
Mushroom: oyster, raw (1 average serving/115g)	0	4
Mushroom: pilau (1 average serving/115g)	21	4
Mushroom: shiitake, dried, cooked (½ cup/50g)	0	1
Mushroom: shiitake, dried, raw (½ cup/12g)	0	2
Mushroom: soup, cream of, canned, made with equal volume of water (1 cup/244g)	22	3
Mushroom: soup, cream of, canned (1 cup/248g)	18	3
Mushroom: soup, cream of, canned, made with equal volume of milk (1 cup/248g)	38	8
Mushroom: soup, dehydrated, made with water (1 cup/253g)	12	5
Mushroom: soup, with barley, canned, made with equal volume of water (1 cup/244g)	5	3
Mushroom: soup, with beef stock, canned, made with equal volume of water (1 cup/244g)	11	4

	RiskPoints ✗	LifePoints ✔
Mushroom: straw, canned, drained (½ cup pieces/78g)	0	1
Mustard: and cress, raw (½ cup/25g)	0	1
Mustard: leaves bhaji (1 average serving/115g)	33	6
Mustard: leaves, boiled (½ cup chopped/70g)	0	2
Mustard: leaves, raw (1 cup chopped/28g)	0	1
Mustard: leaves with spinach bhaji (1 average serving/115g)	33	7
Nori: dried, raw (1 sheet/10g) ☺ DietMentor: Traditionally used to wrap sushi and rice balls, you can simply crumble a sheet on to your soup or salad.	0	11
Okra: bhaji, Bangladeshi, with butter ghee (1 average serving/115g)	33	8
Okra: bhaji, Bangladeshi, with vegetable oil (1 average serving/115g)	18	8
Okra: bhaji, Islami (1 average serving/115g)	47	16
Okra: boiled (½ cup slices/92g)	2	7
Okra: canned (½ cup slices/92g)	1	5
Okra: curry (1 average serving/115g)	25	8
Okra: raw (½ cup slices/50g)	1	5
Okra: stir-fried in corn oil (½ cup slices/92g)	60	12
Okra: with tomatoes and onion, Greek (1 average serving/115g)	48	10

	RiskPoints ✘	LifePoints ✔
Okra: with tomatoes and onion, West Indian (1 average serving/115g)	22	11
Onion: baked (1 large onion/180g) ☺ *DietMentor*: Top and tail each onion, push a whole clove into the top and bake, occasionally basting with a little tomato sauce or vegetable stock.	2	15
Onion: boiled (½ cup chopped/105g)	0	2
Onion: cocktail/silverskin (10 small/55g)	0	0
Onion: dried (¼ cup/14g)	0	1
Onion: fried in corn oil (¼ cup/60g)	16	3
Onion: pakora/bhaji, fried in vegetable oil (1 pakora/25g)	9	3
Onion: pakora/bhaji, retail (1 pakora/25g)	13	2
Onion: pickled (3 medium/75g)	0	1
Onion: raw (1 tbsp chopped/10g)	0	0
Onion: raw (½ cup chopped/80g)	0	3
Onion: ring, breaded and fried (3 rings/30g)	18	1
Onion: sautéed in olive oil (¼ cup/60g)	13	1
Onion: soup, canned, made with equal volume of water (1 cup/241g)	4	3
Onion: soup, cream of, canned, made with equal volume of water (1 cup/244g)	13	2

	RiskPoints ✗	LifePoints ✔
Onion: soup, cream of, made with equal volume of milk (1 cup/248g)	30	9
Onion: soup, dehydrated, made with water (1 cup/246g)	1	1
Onion: spring, bulbs only, raw (½ cup chopped/50g)	0	3
Onion: spring (includes tops and bulb), raw (½ cup chopped/50g)	0	3
Onion: Welsh, raw (½ cup chopped/50g)	0	2
Parsley: freeze-dried (1 tbsp/0.4g)	0	0
Parsley: freeze-dried (¼ cup/1.4g)	0	2
Parsley: raw (½ cup chopped/30g) ☺ *DietMentor*: When used in useful quantities such as this, parsley shows just how green it really is. Add lots, finely chopped, to bulghur salads, yogurt dips or tomato sauces.	0	5
Parsley: raw (10 sprigs/10g)	0	1
Parsnip: boiled (1 parsnip 9 in. long/160g)	4	9
Parsnip: boiled (½ cup slices/78g)	2	4
Parsnip: raw (1 parsnip 9 in. long/160g)	4	14
Parsnip: raw (½ cup slices/67g)	1	6
Patra: leaves, raw (½ cup chopped/28g)	1	3
Pepper: chilli, hot green, raw (1 pepper/45g)	0	4

	RiskPoints ✗	LifePoints ✔
Pepper: chilli, hot red, raw (1 pepper/45g)	0	5
Pepper: green, boiled (1 pepper/74g)	0	3
Pepper: green, boiled (½ cup chopped/68g)	0	2
Pepper: green, raw (1 pepper/74g)	0	4
Pepper: green, raw (½ cup chopped/50g)	0	2
Pepper: jalapeño, canned (½ cup chopped/68g)	1	3
Pepper: red, boiled (1 pepper/74g)	0	4
Pepper: red, boiled (½ cup chopped/68g)	0	4
Pepper: red, raw (1 pepper/74g)	0	5
Pepper: red, raw (½ cup chopped/50g)	0	3
Pepper: stuffed with rice (1 average serving/115g)	6	4
Pepper: stuffed with rice and lamb filling and tomato sauce (1 average serving/115g)	11	7
Pepper: stuffed with vegetable filling and tomato sauce (1 average serving/115g)	11	6
Pepper: stuffed with vegetables, with cheese topping (1 average serving/115g)	19	6
Pepper: yellow, raw (1 pepper/74g)	0	4
Pepper: yellow, raw (½ cup chopped/50g)	0	3
Pepperpot: soup, canned, made with equal volume of water (1 cup/241g)	15	5

	RiskPoints ✘	LifePoints ✔
Pickle: cucumber, sour (1 medium/35g)	0	0
Pickle: cucumber, sweet (1 medium/35g)	0	0
Pickle: cucumber, dill (1 medium/65g)	0	0
Pimiento: canned (1 tbsp/12g)	0	0
Plantain: boiled (½ cup slices/77g)	0	3
Plantain: fried in oil (½ cup slices/80g)	18	7
Plantain: raw (½ cup slices/74g)	0	3
Potato: see potato dishes and products (page 255)		
Pumpkin: boiled (½ cup/122g)	0	3
Pumpkin: canned (½ cup/122g)	1	7
Pumpkin: pie mix, canned (½ cup/135g)	0	9
Purslane: boiled (½ cup/58g)	0	2
Purslane: raw (½ cup/22g)	0	1
Quorn: mycoprotein (1 average serving/115g)	10	17
Radicchio: raw (½ cup shredded/28g)	0	1
Radish: leaves, raw (½ cup shredded/28g)	0	2
Radish: mooli, boiled (½ cup slices/74g)	0	1
Radish: mooli, raw (1 mooli 7 in. long/338g)	0	14
Radish: mooli, raw (½ cup slices/44g)	0	1
Radish: red, raw (½ cup slices/58g)	0	2
Radish: red, raw (10 radishes/45g)	0	1

	RiskPoints ✗	LifePoints ✔
Radish: white icicle, raw (1 radish/17g)	0	0
Radish: white icicle, raw (½ cup slices/50g)	0	1
Rape: leaves, raw (½ cup chopped/28g)	0	1
Ratatouille: made from traditional recipe (½ cup/107g) ☺ *DietMentor*: This is traditionally made with loads of olive oil, hence the RiskPoints.	30	3
Ratatouille: retail (½ cup/107g)	17	4
Salad: carrot and nut with French dressing, retail (1 average serving/115g)	50	7
Salad: Greek (feta cheese, olives and olive oil) (1 average serving/115g)	35	5
Salad: green (lettuce, cucumber, pepper and celery), no dressing (1 average serving/115g)	0	4
Salad: mixed vegetable, no dressing (1 average serving/115g)	0	5
Salad: mixed vegetable, with cheese and egg, no dressing (1 average serving/115g)	11	6
Salad: mixed vegetable, with pasta and seafood, no dressing (1 average serving/115g)	14	7
Salad: mixed vegetable, with shrimp, no dressing (1 average serving/115g)	3	12
Salad: mixed vegetable, with turkey, ham and cheese, no dressing (1 average serving/115g)	21	10
Salad: Waldorf (1 average serving/115g)	50	3

	RiskPoints ✗	LifePoints ✔
Salad: white cabbage, celery and fruit, with mayonnaise, retail (1 average serving/115g)	58	3
Salsify: boiled (½ cup slices/68g)	0	2
Salsify: raw (½ cup slices/67g)	0	3
Sauerkraut: (1 average serving/115g) ☺ *DietMentor*: Don't overlook this one! A little in a sandwich or beside a plate of greens is tasty and irresistible.	0	4
Seakale: boiled (1 average serving/115g)	0	2
Sesbania: flower, steamed (½ cup/52g)	0	2
Shallot: raw (½ cup chopped/80g)	0	3
Shepherd's pie: vegetable (1 average serving/115g)	11	7
Spinach: bhaji (1 average serving/115g)	33	15
Spinach: boiled (½ cup/90g)	1	10
Spinach: canned (½ cup/107g)	1	6
Spinach: curry (1 average serving/115g)	26	9
Spinach: flan (1 average serving/115g)	37	13
Spinach: flan, wholemeal (1 average serving/115g)	37	14
Spinach: frozen, boiled (½ cup/95g)	1	10
Spinach: lasagne (1 average serving/115g)	11	6

	RiskPoints ✗	LifePoints ✔
Spinach: lasagne, wholemeal (1 average serving/115g)	11	8
Spinach: pakora/bhaji, fried in vegetable oil (1 pakora/25g)	13	3
Spinach: pie (1 average serving/115g)	39	15
Spinach: raw (½ cup chopped/28g)	0	4
Spinach: roulade (1 average serving/115g)	64	16
Spinach: soufflé (1 average serving/115g)	45	15
Spinach: with potato bhaji (1 average serving/115g)	40	13
Spinach: with potato curry (1 average serving/115g)	24	7
Spirulina: dried (1 tsp/5g)	0	3
Spring greens: boiled (½ cup chopped/72g)	1	7
Spring greens: raw (½ cup chopped/28g)	0	4
Squash: acorn, baked (½ cup cubes/102g)	0	5
Squash: butternut, baked (½ cup cubes/102g)	0	4
Squash: spaghetti, baked (½ cup/78g)	0	1
Squash: summer crookneck and straightneck, boiled (½ cup slices/90g)	0	3
Squash: winter hubbard, baked (½ cup cubes/102g)	1	5
Swede: boiled (½ cup cubes/85g)	0	2
Sweet potato: baked (1 sweet potato 5 in. long/114g)	1	6

	RiskPoints ✗	LifePoints ✔
Sweet potato: baked (½ cup mashed/100g)	1	5
Sweet potato: boiled (½ cup mashed/164g)	1	7
Sweet potato: candied (1 piece/105g)	10	3
Sweet potato: canned (½ cup/127g)	0	9
Sweet potato: canned, in syrup (½ cup/98g)	0	3
Sweet potato: steamed (1 sweet potato 5 in. long/114g)	0	4
Sweet potato: with green banana, casserole (1 average serving/115g)	36	4
Sweet potato: with onion layer (West Indian) (1 average serving/115g)	14	7
Sweetcorn: baby, fresh and frozen, boiled (½ cup/77g)	0	9
Sweetcorn: boiled (½ cup cut/82g)	4	5
Sweetcorn: boiled (kernels from 1 ear/77g)	2	3
Sweetcorn: canned (½ cup/82g)	0	1
Sweetcorn: canned, cream style (½ cup/128g)	1	6
Sweetcorn: kernels, raw (½ cup cut/77g)	3	5
Sweetcorn: on the cob, with butter (1 ear/146g)	12	9
Tabbouleh: (1 average serving/115g)	13	5
Tannia: raw (½ cup cubes/75g)	0	1
Taro: baked (½ cup cubes/75g)	0	2

	RiskPoints ✗	LifePoints ✔
Taro: boiled (½ cup cubes/75g)	0	2
Taro: leaves, steamed (½ cup/90g)	1	8
Taro: steamed (½ cup cubes/75g)	0	2
Tomato: bisque, canned, made with equal volume of milk (1 cup/251g)	23	10
Tomato: bisque, canned, made with equal volume of water (1 cup/247g)	6	4
Tomato: canned, whole contents (½ cup/120g)	0	3
Tomato: cherry, raw (½ cup chopped/90g)	0	3
Tomato: cherry, raw (6 small/110g)	1	4
Tomato: chutney, home-made (1 tbsp/16g)	0	0
Tomato: chutney, retail (1 tbsp/16g)	0	0
Tomato: fried in corn oil (1 tomato, medium/123g)	23	4
Tomato: grilled (1 average serving/115g)	2	12
Tomato: juice (1 cup/244g)	0	5
Tomato: paste, canned (1 tbsp/16g)	0	1
Tomato: paste, canned (½ cup/131g)	2	15
Tomato: purée (1 tbsp/15g)	0	1
Tomato: purée (½ cup/125g)	0	15
Tomato: raw (1 medium tomato/123g)	0	4
Tomato: raw (½ cup chopped/90g)	0	3

	RiskPoints ✗	LifePoints ✔
Tomato: sauce, canned (½ cup/122g)	0	5
Tomato: sauce, canned, Spanish style (½ cup/122g)	0	7
Tomato: sauce, canned, with herbs and cheese (½ cup/122g)	5	5
Tomato: sauce, canned, with mushrooms (½ cup/122g)	0	5
Tomato: sauce canned, with onions (½ cup/122g)	0	7
Tomato: sauce, canned, with onions, green peppers and celery (½ cup/122g)	2	6
Tomato: sauce, canned, with tomato tidbits (½ cup/122g)	1	5
Tomato: soup, canned, made with equal volume of milk (1 cup/248g)	21	11
Tomato: soup, canned, made with equal volume of water (1 cup/244g)	4	5
Tomato: soup, cream of, canned (1 cup/244g)	18	5
Tomato: soup, dehydrated, made with water (1 cup/265g)	8	3
Tomato: soup, with rice, canned, made with equal volume of water (1 cup/247g)	6	4
Tomato: soup, with vegetables, dehydrated, made with water (1 cup/253g)	2	2
Tomato: stewed (½ cup/51g)	3	2
Tomato: stuffed with rice (1 average serving/115g)	38	4
Tomato: stuffed with vegetables (1 average serving/115g)	17	6

	RiskPoints ✗	LifePoints ✔
Tomato: sun-dried (1 piece/2g)	0	0
Tomato: sun-dried (½ cup/27g)	2	7
Tomato: sun-dried, packed in oil (1 piece/3g)	1	0
Tomato: sun-dried, packed in oil (½ cup/55g)	19	7
Tomato: with onion salad (1 average serving/115g)	17	4
Turnip: bhaji, made with butter (1 average serving/115g)	93	4
Turnip: boiled in salted water (½ cup cubes/78g)	0	1
Turnip: boiled in salted water (½ cup mashed/115g)	0	2
Turnip: raw (½ cup cubes/65g) ☺ DietMentor: Grate one of these into a winter salad for a fresh, crunchy taste.	0	2
Turnip: tops, boiled (½ cup chopped/72g)	0	11
Turnip: with onion bhaji (1 average serving/115g)	31	3
Vegetable bake: mixed vegetables topped with cheese sauce and breadcrumbs (1 average serving/115g)	25	7
Vegetable banger: made up with water (1 banger/30g)	5	3
Vegetable banger: made up with water and egg (1 banger/30g)	6	3
Vegetable banger: made up with water and egg, fried in sunflower oil (1 banger/30g)	13	3

	RiskPoints ✗	LifePoints ✔
Vegetable banger: made up with water and egg, fried in vegetable oil (1 banger/30g)	13	3
Vegetable banger: made up with water, fried in sunflower oil (1 banger/30g)	11	2
Vegetable banger: made up with water, fried in vegetable oil (1 banger/30g)	11	2
Vegetable bhaji: Punjabi, with butter (1 average serving/115g)	37	9
Vegetable bhaji: Pubjabi, with vegetable oil (1 average serving/115g)	24	9
Vegetable bhaji: with butter (1 average serving/115g)	84	7
Vegetable bhaji: with vegetable oil (1 average serving/115g)	53	6
Vegetable burger: in bun, with lettuce, tomato and ketchup (1 burger/176g)	17	18
Vegetable burger: made up with water (1 burger/70g)	8	12
Vegetable burger: made up with water and egg (1 burger/70g)	10	12
Vegetable burger: made up with water and egg, fried in sunflower oil (1 burger/70g)	22	11
Vegetable burger: made up with water and egg, fried in vegetable oil (1 burger/70g)	22	11
Vegetable burger: made up with water and egg, grilled (1 burger/70g)	11	11
Vegetable burger: made up with water, fried in sunflower oil (1 burger/70g)	20	10

	RiskPoints ✗	LifePoints ✔
Vegetable burger: made up with water, fried in vegetable oil (1 burger/70g)	20	10
Vegetable burger: made up with water, grilled (1 burger/70g)	9	10
Vegetable burger: Tivall low-fat, chargrilled (1 burger/75g)	9	26
Vegetable casserole: (1 average serving/115g)	1	6
Vegetable chilli: (1 average serving/115g)	1	5
Vegetable chilli: retail (1 average serving/115g)	6	6
Vegetable crumble: in milk base (1 average serving/115g)	25	7
Vegetable crumble: in milk base, wholemeal (1 average serving/115g)	26	9
Vegetable crumble: in tomato base (1 average serving/115g)	29	6
Vegetable crumble: in tomato base, wholemeal (1 average serving/115g)	30	8
Vegetable curry: in sweet sauce (1 average serving/115g)	6	4
Vegetable curry: Islami (1 average serving/115g)	12	6
Vegetable curry: made with frozen mixed vegetables (1 average serving/115g)	17	5
Vegetable curry: Pakistani (1 average serving/115g)	7	6
Vegetable curry: retail, with rice (1 average serving/115g)	8	4
Vegetable curry: takeaway (1 average serving/115g)	21	2

	RiskPoints ✗	LifePoints ✔
Vegetable curry: West Indian (1 average serving/115g)	11	9
Vegetable curry: with yogurt (1 average serving/115g)	11	6
Vegetable flan: (1 average serving/115g)	37	7
Vegetable flan: wholemeal (1 average serving/115g)	37	9
Vegetable juice: cocktail (1 cup/242g)	0	9
☺ *DietMentor*: Add a dash of shoyu soy sauce or a pinch of black pepper for extra tang.		
Vegetable lasagne: (1 average serving/115g)	18	5
Vegetable lasagne: retail (1 average serving/115g)	15	10
Vegetable lasagne: wholemeal (1 average serving/115g)	18	7
Vegetable moussaka: (1 average serving/115g)	27	6
Vegetable pakora/bhaji: retail (1 pakora/25g)	9	2
Vegetable pasty: (1 average serving/115g)	42	5
Vegetable pasty: wholemeal (1 average serving/115g)	43	9
Vegetable pie: (1 average serving/115g)	21	6
Vegetable pie: wholemeal (1 average serving/115g)	22	8
Vegetable pilau: (1 average serving/115g)	20	4
Vegetable purée: (1 tbsp/15g)	1	0

	RiskPoints ✗	LifePoints ✔
Vegetable purée: (½ cup/125g)	13	5
Vegetable rissoles: fried in sunflower oil (2 rissoles/120g)	21	4
Vegetable rissoles: fried in vegetable oil (2 rissoles/120g)	21	4
Vegetable salad: canned (1 average serving/115g)	28	3
Vegetable samosa: retail (1 average serving/115g)	26	8
Vegetable soup: canned (1 cup/240g)	3	7
Vegetable soup: canned, chunky (1 cup/240g)	9	8
Vegetable soup: canned, made with equal volume of water (1 cup/241g)	4	4
Vegetable soup: cream of, dehydrated, made with water (1 cup/260g)	14	10
Vegetable soup: home-made (1 cup/250g)	48	5
Vegetable soup: with beef broth, canned, made with equal volume of water (1 cup/241g)	4	4
Vegetable stir-fry mix: fried in corn oil (1 average serving/115g)	10	5
Vegetable stir-fry mix: fried in sunflower oil (1 average serving/115g)	10	5
Vegetable stir-fry mix: fried in vegetable oil (1 average serving/115g)	10	5
Vegetable stock cube: (1 cube/5g)	2	0
Vegetables mixed: canned, reheated, drained (1 average serving/115g)	2	3

	RiskPoints ✗	LifePoints ✔
Vegetables mixed: frozen, boiled (1 average serving/115g)	1	8
Vegetables: stir-fry type, frozen, fried in blended oil (1 average serving/115g)	10	5
Vine leaves: stuffed with rice (1 average serving/115g)	51	6
Wakame: dried, raw (1 cup/30g)	1	8
Water chestnuts: canned (½ cup slices/70g)	0	1
Watercress: raw (½ cup chopped/17g)	0	1
Yam: baked (½ cup cubes/68g)	0	3
Yam: boiled (½ cup cubes/68g)	0	2
Yam: steamed (½ cup cubes/68g)	0	2
Yeast: baker's, compressed (1 tbsp/30g)	0	17
Yeast: dried (2 tbsp/30g)	1	31
Yeast: extract (1 tsp/5g)	0	10
Yeast: extract (1 tbsp/15g)	0	27
Yeast: extract, fortified with vitamin B12 (1 tsp/5g) ☺ DietMentor: We use this as the basis for our LifePoints Sauté: a no-fat, aromatic sauté method that will have your mouth watering.	0	11
Yeast: extract, fortified with vitamin B12 (1 tbsp/15g)	0	31

Potato Dishes & Products

Chips: crinkle-cut, frozen, fried in corn oil (regular order/75g)	31	6
Chips: fine-cut, frozen, fried in corn oil (regular order/75g)	39	7

	RiskPoints ✗	LifePoints ✔
Chips: French fries, retail (regular order/75g)	29	4
Chips: home-made, fried in corn oil (regular order/75g)	12	6
Chips: microwave, cooked (regular order/75g)	18	5
Chips: oven, frozen, baked (regular order/75g)	7	5
Chips: oven, thick-cut, frozen, baked (regular order/75g)	8	5
Chips: retail, fried in vegetable oil (regular order/75g)	23	3
Chips: straight-cut, frozen, fried in corn oil (regular order/75g)	25	6
Chips: thick-cut, frozen, fried in corn oil (regular order/75g)	19	6
Crisps: average (1 bag/25g)	26	3
Crisps: crinkle-cut (1 bag/25g)	27	3
Crisps: jacket (1 bag/25g)	24	3
Crisps: low-fat (1 bag/25g)	17	3
Crisps: square (1 bag/25g)	16	1
Crisps: thick, crinkle-cut (1 bag/25g)	23	3
Crisps: thick-cut (1 bag/25g)	21	3
Duchesse potatoes: (1 average serving/115g)	25	6
Instant potato powder: made up with semi-skimmed milk (½ cup/105g)	1	4
Instant potato powder: made up with skimmed milk (½ cup/105g)	0	4
Instant potato powder: made up with water (½ cup/105g)	0	3

	RiskPoints ✘	LifePoints ✔
Instant potato powder: made up with whole milk (½ cup/105g)	3	4
New potato: boiled (3 potatoes/150g)	1	6
New Potato: canned (3 potatoes/150g)	0	5
New potato: chipped, fried in corn oil (3 potatoes/150g)	35	9
New potato: frozen, 'roast' in corn oil (3 potatoes/150g)	24	6
Old potato: baked, flesh and skin (1 medium/156g)	0	15
Old potato: baked, flesh only (1 medium/140g)	0	8
Old potato: boiled (1 medium/150g)	0	8
Old potato: mashed (1 medium/150g)	16	8
Old potato: mashed (½ cup/78g)	8	4
Old potato: roast in corn oil (1 medium/150g)	16	10
Potato and corn stick snacks: (1 pack/25g)	14	2
Potato: and leek soup (1 cup/250g)	30	7
Potato: and tapioca snacks (1 pack/25g)	15	2
Potato: bhaji, with butter ghee (1 average serving/115g)	55	6
Potato: bhaji, with vegetable oil (1 average serving/115g)	28	6
Potato: cakes, fried in lard (1 average serving/115g)	33	6
Potato: cakes, fried in vegetable oil (1 average serving/115g)	24	6

	RiskPoints ✗	LifePoints ✓
Potato: carrot and pea pakora/ bhaji, fried in vegetable oil (1 pakora/25g)	14	3
Potato: croquettes, fried in blended oil (1 average serving/115g)	37	5
Potato: curry, Bombay (1 average serving/115g)	19	5
Potato: curry, Gujerati (1 average serving/115g)	15	3
Potato: curry, Punjabi (1 average serving/115g)	21	5
Potato: flour (½ cup/90g)	2	5
Potato: leek and celery bake (1 average serving/115g)	33	6
Potato: onion and mushroom bhaji (1 average serving/115g)	50	6
Potato: pakora/bhaji, fried in vegetable oil (1 pakora/25g)	12	2
Potato: rings, snack type (1 pack/25g)	26	0
Potato: salad, with French dressing (1 average serving/115g)	32	5
Potato: salad, with mayonnaise (1 average serving/115g)	59	5
Potato: salad, with mayonnaise, retail (1 average serving/115g)	76	5
Potato: salad, with reduced-calorie dressing, retail (1 average serving/115g)	11	4
Potato: spinach and cauliflower (1 average serving/115g)	83	7
Potato: waffles, frozen, cooked (1 waffle/35g)	7	0

	RiskPoints ✗	LifePoints ✓
Potato: with cauliflower pakora/ bhaji, fried in vegetable oil (1 pakora/25g)	13	2
Potato: with fenugreek leaves bhaji (1 average serving/115g)	45	8
Potato: with green pepper bhaji (1 average serving/115g)	26	5
Potato: with onion bhaji (1 average serving/115g)	56	6
Potato: with pea curry (1 average serving/115g)	10	6
Potato: with eggs (Greek: fried potatoes with onion and egg) (1 average serving/115g)	68	14
Puffed potato snack products: (1 pack/25g)	20	1

GROUP FOUR: LEGUMES, NUTS & SEEDS

Legumes & Beans

	RiskPoints ✗	LifePoints ✔
Aduki bean: boiled (½ cup/115g) ☺ *DietMentor*: Kids love these little 'pink peas' served on rice or couscous.	0	7
Alfalfa: sprouts, raw (½ cup/16g)	0	0
Baked bean: Asda Healthy Choice, lower in sugar and salt (average serving/215g)	2	14
Baked bean: canned, in tomato sauce (average serving/215g)	3	14
Baked bean: canned, in tomato sauce, with burgers (average serving/215g)	15	13
Baked bean: canned, in tomato sauce, with pork sausages (average serving/215g)	24	12
Baked bean: canned, with beef (average serving/215g)	27	14
Baked bean: canned, with pork (average serving/215g)	9	15
Baked bean: home-made (average serving/215g)	31	17
Baked bean: on toast (½ can beans on 1 slice toast with no butter or margarine/233g)	4	17
Baked bean: on toast, with butter (½ can beans on 1 slice toast with butter/238g)	22	17
Balor bean: canned (½ cup/115g)	0	2
Barbecue beans: canned, in sauce (average serving/215g)	2	7
Bean: and lentil chilli (1 average serving/115g)	7	7

	RiskPoints ✗	LifePoints ✔
Bean: and mixed vegetable casserole (1 average serving/115g)	2	6
Bean: and root vegetable casserole (1 average serving/115g)	1	5
Bean: salad, retail (1 average serving/115g)	26	7
Bean: soup with bacon, dehydrated, made with water (1 cup/265g)	7	6
Bean: soup with frankfurters, canned, made with equal volume of water (1 cup/250g)	17	8
Bean: soup with ham, canned, chunky, ready to serve (1 cup/243g)	24	13
Bean: soup with pork, canned, made with equal volume of water (1 cup/253g)	14	8
Bean sprouts: mung beans, boiled (½ cup/62g)	0	2
Bean sprouts: mung beans, canned (½ cup/62g)	0	1
Bean sprouts: mung beans, raw (½ cup/52g)	0	3
Bean sprouts: mung beans, stir-fried (½ cup/62g)	0	5
Black bean: boiled (½ cup/86g) ☺ DietMentor: Cook until very soft, then add grated ginger and garlic and serve hot over rice.	1	11
Black bean: soup, canned, made with equal volume of water (1 cup/247g)	3	7
Black gram: chilki urad dhal, boiled (1 average serving/115g)	1	7

	RiskPoints ✗	LifePoints ✔
Black gram: curry, Bengali (1 average serving/115g)	14	4
Black gram: curry, Gujerati (1 average serving/115g)	35	9
Black gram: curry, with kidney beans (1 average serving/115g)	14	5
Black gram: dhal (1 average serving/115g)	18	4
Black gram: duhli urad dhal, boiled (1 average serving/115g)	1	8
Black gram: urad gram, boiled (1 average serving/115g)	1	8
Blackeye bean: boiled (½ cup/86g) ☺ DietMentor: These are stunning stirred into a salad.	1	12
Blackeye bean: curry, Gujerati (1 average serving/115g)	12	10
Blackeye bean: curry, Punjabi (1 average serving/115g)	21	12
Broad bean: boiled (½ cup/85g) ☺ DietMentor: Boiled or steamed with fresh mint is a traditional preparation, hot or cold.	1	5
Broad bean: canned (½ cup/85g)	1	6
Broad bean: frozen, boiled (½ cup/85g)	1	6
Broad bean: boiled (½ cup/80g)	1	4
Butter bean: canned (½ cup/80g)	1	2
Chevda/chevraic hewra: (spiced lentils with peanuts) (1 average serving/115g)	92	20
Chick pea: boiled (½ cup/82g)	4	7

	RiskPoints ✗	LifePoints ✔
Chick pea: canned (½ cup/82g)	5	3
Chick pea: curry (1 average serving/115g)	21	12
Chick pea: dhal (1 average serving/115g)	17	9
Chick pea: dhal and spinach, with butter (1 average serving/115g)	59	9
Chick pea: dhal and spinach, with vegetable oil (1 average serving/115g)	40	9
Chick pea: flour/besan flour (½ cup/90g)	12	26
Chick pea: rissoles, fried in sunflower oil (2 rissoles/120g)	50	7
Chick pea: rissoles, fried in vegetable oil (2 rissoles/120g)	50	14
Chick pea: with potato curry (1 average serving/115g)	15	6
Chick pea: with tomato curry, Gujerati, with butter ghee (1 average serving/115g)	73	11
Chick pea: with tomato curry, Gujerati, with vegetable oil (1 average serving/115g)	41	10
Chick pea: with tomato curry, Punjabi, with butter (1 average serving/115g)	17	7
Chick pea: with tomato curry, Punjabi, with vegetable oil (1 average serving/115g)	14	7
Chilli bean: canned, reheated (1 average serving/215g)	2	9
Cluster bean: raw (½ cup/55g)	0	3
Cowpea: catjang, boiled (½ cup/86g)	1	11

	RiskPoints ✗	LifePoints ✔
Cowpea: common (black-eyed crowder southern), boiled (½ cup/86g)	1	13
Cowpea: common (black-eyed crowder southern), canned (½ cup/120g)	1	7
Cowpea: common (black-eyed crowder southern), canned, with pork (½ cup/120g)	5	7
Dhal: Dhokari (1 average serving/115g)	9	7
Dhal: made with mung beans (1 average serving/115g)	11	6
Dudhi kofta: Gujerati (1 average serving/115g)	21	5
French bean: *see* 'Green bean'		
Green bean: bhaji (1 average serving/115g)	21	6
Green bean: curry (1 average serving/115g)	36	5
Green bean: boiled (½ cup/62g) ☺ *DietMentor*: Irresistible freshly cooked and stirred into a salad or sprinkled with black pepper and a squeeze of lemon.	0	3
Green bean: canned (½ cup/68g)	0	2
Green bean: frozen, boiled (½ cup/62g)	0	3
Haricot bean: boiled (½ cup/85g)	1	5
Hyacinth-bean: boiled (½ cup/44g)	0	2
Khatiyu: Gujerati (1 average serving/115g)	20	7
Khichadi: with butter ghee (1 average serving/115g)	25	5

	RiskPoints ✗	LifePoints ✔
Khichadi: with vegetable oil (1 average serving/115g)	14	5
Kidney bean: curry, Gujerati (1 average serving/115g)	17	5
Kidney bean: curry, Punjabi (1 average serving/115g)	16	6
Kidney bean: with mung bean curry (1 average serving/115g)	34	4
Kidney bean: red, boiled (½ cup/88g)	1	8
Kidney bean: red, canned (½ cup/128g)	1	9
Lentil: and cheese pie (1 average serving/115g)	34	12
Lentil: and potato pie (1 average serving/115g)	6	7
Lentil: and tomato flan (1 average serving/115g)	18	8
Lentil: and tomato flan, wholemeal (1 average serving/115g)	18	10
Lentil: curry, red/masoor dhal and mung bean dhal (1 average serving/115g)	19	4
Lentil: curry, red/masoor dhal and tomato, Punjabi (1 average serving/115g)	15	4
Lentil: curry, red/masoor dhal and tomato, with butter (1 average serving/115g)	26	4
Lentil: curry, red/masoor dhal and tomato, with vegetable oil (1 average serving/115g)	16	4
Lentil: curry, red/masoor dhal and vegetable (1 average serving/115g)	10	7

	RiskPoints ✗	LifePoints ✔
Lentil: curry, red/masoor dhal, mung bean dhal and tomato (1 average serving/115g)	12	4
Lentil: curry, red/masoor dhal, Punjabi (1 average serving/115g)	13	8
Lentil: curry, red/masoor dhal with butter (1 average serving/115g)	34	8
Lentil: curry, red/masoor dhal, with vegetable oil (1 average serving/115g)	22	8
Lentil: curry, whole/masoor, Gujerati (1 average serving/115g)	28	8
Lentil: curry, whole/masoor, Punjabi (1 average serving/115g)	24	7
Lentil: green and brown, boiled (½ cup/99g) ☺ DietMentor: These are also called continental lentils.	1	8
Lentil: pie (1 average serving/115g)	12	10
Lentil: red, canned, in tomato sauce (1 average serving/115g)	0	4
Lentil: red, split boiled (½ cup/98g ☺ DietMentor: Keep bags of these on hand, they need no soaking and are very quick to cook. They are the basis of most lentil soups, loaves, cutlets and spreads. Kids love them!	0	5
Lentil: rissoles, fried in sunflower oil (2 rissoles/120g)	31	12
Lentil: rissoles, fried in vegetable oil (2 rissoles/120g)	31	12

	RiskPoints ✗	LifePoints ✔
Lentil: soup, canned (1 cup/240g)	1	7
Lentil: soup, home-made (1 cup/240g)	54	11
Lentil: soup with ham, canned, ready to serve (1 cup/248g)	8	11
Lentil: sprouted, raw (½ cup/38g)	0	5
Lentil: sprouted, stir-fried (½ cup/45g)	0	2
Lilva: bean, canned (½ cup/128g)	1	10
Mange-tout: boiled in salted water (½ cup/80g)	0	4
Mange-tout: raw (½ cup/72g)	0	5
Mulligatawny: soup (1 cup/245g)	67	7
Mung: bean and turnip leaves curry (1 average serving/115g)	40	10
Mung: bean, boiled (½ cup/101g)	1	7
Mung: bean curry, Gujerati (1 average serving/115g)	16	6
Mung: bean curry, Punjabi (1 average serving/115g)	14	4
Mung: bean dhal and spinach (1 average serving/115g)	8	15
Mung: bean dhal and tomato (1 average serving/115g)	10	5
Mung: bean dhal, Bengali (1 average serving/115g)	18	3
Mung: bean dhal, Punjabi (1 average serving/115g)	8	6
Navy bean: boiled (½ cup/91g)	1	12
Navy bean: canned (½ cup/131g)	1	12
Papri bean: canned (½ cup/101g)	0	4

	RiskPoints ✗	LifePoints ✔
Pea: and potato curry (1 average serving/115g)	31	4
Pea: bhaji, made with butter (1 average serving/115g)	188	10
Pea: boiled (½ cup/80g)	3	9
Pea: canned (½ cup/85g)	1	5
Pea: dried, boiled (½ cup/80g)	1	4
Pea: frozen, boiled (½ cup/80g)	1	8
Pea: green, soup, canned, made with equal volume of milk (1 cup/254g)	30	12
Pea: green, soup, canned, made with equal volume of water (1 cup/250g)	10	6
Pea: green, soup, dehydrated, made with water (1 cup/271g)	3	9
Pea: marrowfat, Asda Healthy Choice (low sugar and salt) (½ cup/75g)	1	4
Pea: marrowfat, canned (½ cup/75g)	1	3
Pea: mushy, canned (½ cup/120g)	2	2
Pea: petits pois, canned (½ cup/85g)	1	6
Pea: petits pois, frozen, boiled (½ cup/80g)	1	7
Pea: processed, canned (½ cup/110g)	1	6
Pea: raw (½ cup/72g)	2	10
☺ *DietMentor*: Yes! If you grow these yourself you will already know how sweet and crunchy raw peas are. Now, can you stop eating them or there won't be any left for the pot!		

	RiskPoints ✗	LifePoints ✔
Pea: split, boiled (½ cup/98g)	0	8
Pea: split, soup with ham, canned, chunky, ready to serve (1 cup/240g)	11	11
Pea: split, soup with ham, canned, made with equal volume of water (1 cup/253g)	13	7
Pea: sugar-snap, boiled (½ cup/75g)	0	3
Pea: sugar-snap, raw (½ cup/68g)	0	4
Pea: with carrots, canned (½ cup/128g)	0	7
Pea: with carrots, frozen, boiled (½ cup/80g)	0	6
Pea: with onions, canned (½ cup/60g)	0	3
Pea: with onions, frozen, boiled (½ cup/90g)	0	4
Pease pudding: canned (1 average serving/115g)	1	1
Pigeon pea: boiled (½ cup/84g)	1	5
Pigeon pea: dhal and tomato (1 average serving/115g)	6	2
Pigeon pea: dhal, boiled (1 average serving/115g)	1	7
Pigeon pea: dhal, with butter (1 average serving/115g)	23	4
Pigeon pea: dhal, with vegetable oil (1 average serving/115g)	15	4
Pinto bean: boiled (½ cup/85g)	1	11
Pinto bean: canned (½ cup/120g)	0	9
Refried beans: (1 average serving/115g)	37	12
☺ DietMentor: Traditionally made from pinto beans and lard, hence the high RiskPoints.		

	RiskPoints ✗	LifePoints ✔
Runner beans: boiled (½ cup/62g)	0	2
Soya bean: boiled (½ cup/86g)	15	9
Soya bean: sprouted, raw (½ cup/35g)	5	6
Soya bean: sprouted, steamed (½ cup/47g)	5	4
Soya bean: sprouted, stir-fried (½ cup/50g)	8	8

Legume & Bean Products

Aduki beanburger: fried in vegetable oil (1 burger/70g)	12	5
Bacon: meatless (1 strip/8g)	5	3
Bacon: meatless (½ cup/72g)	53	18
Bean: loaf (1 average serving/115g)	20	9
Bean: pâté, made with lentils (1 average serving/115g) ☺ DietMentor: See our recipe in LifePoints Cookbook and adjust the spices to suit your own taste.	1	16
Black bean: sauce (1 cup/272g)	14	23
Butter bean beanburger: fried in vegetable oil (1 burger/70g)	18	6
Carob: flour (½ cup/51g)	0	6
Dosa: plain (1 average serving/115g)	24	8
Falafel: fried in vegetable oil (3 patties/51g)	14	4
Ganthia: see 'Sev'		
Hummus: (1 average serving/115g)	36	6

	RiskPoints ✗	LifePoints ✔
Kidney bean beanburger: fried in vegetable oil (1 burger/70g)	18	7
Lentil: and nut roast (1 average serving/115g)	34	11
Lentil: and nut roast, with egg (1 average serving/115g)	34	12
Lentil: and rice roast (1 average serving/115g)	5	4
Lentil: and rice roast, with egg (1 average serving/115g)	6	5
Lentil: cutlets, fried in vegetable oil (1 cutlet/88g)	17	7
Lentil: roast (1 average serving/115g)	8	9
Lentil: roast, with egg (1 average serving/115g)	10	10
Miso: (1 tbsp/20g) ☺ DietMentor: This is a paste of fermented soya beans and is delicious added to soups, sauces and stews. Or spread a little on your toast for a savoury wake-up.	3	2
Miso: (½ cup/138g)	20	16
Natto: (½ cup/88g)	24	13
Red pea loaf: (West Indian: made with kidney beans) (1 average serving/115g)	10	11
Sausage: meatless (1 link/25g)	11	9
Sev: (extruded chick pea flour snack) (average serving/30g)	18	6
Soya beanburger: fried in vegetable oil (1 burger/70g)	19	7
Soya milk: (1 cup/240g)	11	7

	RiskPoints ✗	LifePoints ✔
Soya mince: granules (100g) ☺ *DietMentor*: Also known as TVP, texturized vegetable protein, used instead of beef or lamb mince in your favourite dishes.	13	29
Soy sauce: made from soya and wheat (shoyu) (1 tbsp/18g)	0	1
Soy sauce: made from soya and wheat (shoyu) (¼ cup/58g)	0	3
Tempeh: (1 average serving/115g)	18	28
Tempeh burgers: made with rice, fried in vegetable oil (1 burger/70g)	14	5
Tofu burger: baked (1 burger/70g)	7	7
Tofu: dried-frozen (koyadofu) (1 piece/17g)	12	5
Tofu: dried-frozen (koyadofu), prepared with calcium sulphate (1 piece/17g)	12	8
Tofu: fried (1 piece/13g)	6	1
Tofu: fried, prepared with calcium sulphate (1 piece/13g)	6	2
Tofu: fujuk (1 piece/13g)	5	1
Tofu: okara (½ cup/61g)	2	2
Tofu: raw, firm (½ cup/126g)	27	18
Tofu: raw, firm, prepared with calcium sulphate (½ cup/126g)	27	23
Tofu: raw, regular (½ cup/124g)	14	9
Tofu: raw, regular, prepared with calcium sulphate (½ cup/124g)	14	12
Tofu: salted and fermented (fuyu) (1 block/11g)	2	0

	RiskPoints ✗	LifePoints ✔
Tofu: salted and fermented (fuyu), prepared with calcium sulphate (1 block/11g)	2	2
Tofu: soya bean, steamed (½ cup/124g)	13	11
Tofu: soya bean, steamed, fried (½ cup/124g)	54	19
Tofu: spread (1 tbsp/15g)	7	0
TVP: see 'Soya mince'		
Vegetarian drumsticks: Tivall (1 drumstick/50g)	7	17
Vegetarian pâté: retail (soya, cereal and vegetable based) (1 tbsp/15g)	5	5

Nuts & Nut Products

	RiskPoints ✗	LifePoints ✔
Almond: butter (1 tbsp/16g)	23	3
Almond: curry (1 average serving/115g)	136	8
Almond: dried, blanched (1 oz/28g)	37	5
Almond: dried, unblanched (1 oz, 24 whole kernels/28g)	37	6
Almond: dry roasted, unblanched (1 oz/28g)	36	6
Almond: honey roasted, unblanched (1 oz/28g)	35	5
Almond: oil roasted, blanched (1 oz, 24 whole kernels/28g)	40	5
Almond: oil roasted, unblanched (1 oz, 22 whole kernels/28g)	40	7
Almond: paste (1 oz/28g)	19	5
Almond: toasted, unblanched (1 oz/28g)	36	6
Beechnut: dried (1 oz/28g)	35	4

	RiskPoints ✗	LifePoints ✔
Brazil nut: dried, unblanched (1 oz, 6 – 8 kernels/28g)	47	5
Cashew: butter, plain (1 tbsp/16g)	19	2
Cashew: dry roasted (1 oz/28g)	32	5
Cashew: oil roasted (1 oz/28g)	34	5
Chestnut: Chinese, boiled and steamed (1 oz/28g)	0	2
Chestnut: Chinese, roasted (1 oz/28g)	0	3
Chestnut: European, boiled and steamed (1 oz/28g) ☺ *DietMentor*: Mash these, spice them to taste and spread on your toast or rice cake.	0	2
Chestnut: European, roasted (1 oz/28g)	1	3
Chestnut: Japanese, boiled and steamed (1 oz/28g)	0	1
Chestnut: Japanese, roasted (1 oz/28g)	0	3
Coconut: cream, canned (liquid expressed from grated meat) (1 tbsp/19g)	22	0
Coconut: meat, dried (desiccated), creamed (1 oz/28g)	130	2
Coconut: meat, dried (desiccated), sweetened, (½ cup/shredded 46g)	108	2
Coconut: meat, dried (desiccated), toasted (1 oz/28g)	88	2
Coconut: meat, raw (½ cup grated/40g)	89	2
Coconut: milk, canned (liquid expressed from grated meat and water) (1 tbsp/15g)	21	0

	RiskPoints ✗	LifePoints ✔
Coconut: water (liquid from coconuts) (1 cup/240g)	3	3
Coconut: water (liquid from coconuts) (1 tbsp/15g)	0	0
Filbert: see 'Hazelnut'		
Ginkgo nut: canned (1 oz, 14 medium kernels/28g)	1	2
Ginkgo nut: dried (1 oz/28g)	1	6
Ginkgo nut: raw (1 oz/28g)	1	3
Hazelnut: dried, blanched (1 oz/28g)	47	5
Hazelnut: dried, unblanched (1 oz/28g)	44	5
Hazelnut: dry roasted, unblanched (1 oz/28g)	47	5
Hazelnut: oil roasted, unblanched (1 oz/28g)	45	5
Macadamia nut: dried (1 oz/28g)	52	3
Macadamia nut: oil roasted (1 oz, 10 – 12 kernels/28g)	54	2
Mixed nuts: with peanuts, dry roasted (1 oz/28g)	36	5
Mixed nuts: with peanuts, oil roasted (1 oz/28g)	39	6
Mixed nuts: without peanuts, oil roasted (1 oz/28g)	39	5
Nut: and rice roast (1 average serving/115g)	64	13
Nut: and rice roast, with egg (1 average serving/115g)	62	14
Nut: and seed roast (1 average serving/115g)	71	16
Nut: and seed roast, with egg (1 average serving/115g)	68	17

	RiskPoints ✗	LifePoints ✔
Nut: and vegetable roast (1 average serving/115g)	62	14
Nut: and vegetable roast, with egg (1 average serving/115g)	60	15
Nut: croquettes, fried in sunflower oil (1 average serving/115g)	75	11
Nut: croquettes, fried in vegetable oil (1 average serving/115g)	75	11
Nut: cutlets, fried in vegetable oil (1 cutlet/88g)	49	5
Nut: cutlets, grilled (1 cutlet/88g)	28	5
Nut: cutlets, retail, fried in sunflower oil (1 cutlet/88g)	49	5
Nut: mushroom and rice roast (1 average serving/115g)	43	10
Nut: roast (1 average serving/115g)	73	15
Nut: roast, with egg (1 average serving/115g)	71	16
Peanut: butter (1 tbsp/16g)	19	3
Peanut: butter (½ cup/129g)	161	26
Peanut: butter and banana sandwich (1 sandwich/201g) ☺ *DietMentor*: You may not need these, but they are great for kids.	51	21
Peanut: butter and jam sandwich (1 sandwich/127g)	50	15
Peanut: dry roasted (1 oz/28g)	31	9
Peanut: flour, defatted (1 tbsp/4g)	0	1
Peanut: flour, defatted (½ cup/30g)	0	12
Peanut: kernels, oil roasted (1 oz/28g)	35	8

	RiskPoints ✗	LifePoints ✔
Pecan: dried (1 oz/28g)	48	4
Pecan: dry roasted (1 oz/28g)	45	3
Pecan: oil roasted (1 oz, 15 halves/28g)	50	3
Pine nut: pignolia, dried (1 oz, 15 kernels/28g)	35	6
Pine nut: pinyon, dried (1 oz/28g)	43	6
Pistachio nut: dried (1 oz/28g)	34	6
Pistachio: dry roasted (1 oz/28g)	37	4
Pumpkin: and squash seed kernels, dried (1 oz, 142 kernels/28g)	32	7
Pumpkin: and squash seed kernels roasted (1 oz/28g)	29	7
Pumpkin: and squash seeds, whole roasted (1 oz, 85 seeds/28g)	13	3
Sesame: butter paste (1 oz/28g)	36	12
Sesame: flour, partially defatted (½ cup/40g)	11	19
Sesame: seed kernels, dried (1 tbsp/8g)	10	2
Sesame: seed kernels, toasted (1 oz/28g)	34	10
Sesame: seeds, whole dried (1 tbsp/9g)	11	4
Sesame: seeds, whole roasted and toasted (1 oz/28g)	34	12
Sunflower: seed butter (1 tbsp/16g)	19	5
Sunflower: seed flour, partially defatted (½ cup/40g)	1	22
Sunflower: seed kernels, dried (1 oz/28g)	35	13

	RiskPoints ✗	LifePoints ✔
Sunflower: seed kernels, dry roasted (1 oz/28g)	35	9
Sunflower: seed kernels, oil roasted (1 oz/28g)	40	9
Sunflower: seed kernels, toasted (1 oz/28g)	40	9
Tahini: from raw and stone ground sesame kernels (1 tbsp/15g)	18	5
Tahini: from roasted and toasted sesame kernels (most common type) (1 tbsp/15g)	20	5
Tahini: from unroasted sesame kernels (non-chemical removal of seed coat) (1 tbsp/14g)	19	5
Walnut: black, dried (1 oz/28g)	40	4
Walnut: English or Persian, dried (1 oz/28g)	43	4
Watermelon: seed kernels, dried (1 oz/28g)	33	6

MEAT
Beef

	RiskPoints ✗	LifePoints ✔
All cuts: trimmed, lean and fat, cooked (85g)	54	20
All cuts: trimmed, lean, cooked (85g)	24	22
Brisket: lean and fat, braised (85g)	78	18
Brisket: lean only, braised (85g)	29	21
Burger: cheeseburger: 1 large double patty with condiments and vegetables (258g)	132	36
Burger: cheeseburger: 1 large single patty with bacon and condiments (195g)	121	32
Burger: cheeseburger: 1 large single patty with condiments and vegetables (219g)	112	31
Burger: cheeseburger: 1 large single patty with ham, condiments and vegetables (254g)	158	39
Burger: cheeseburger: 1 large single patty, plain (185g)	111	35
Burger: hamburger: 1 large double patty with condiments and vegetables (226g)	78	33
Burger: hamburger: 1 large single patty, with condiments and vegetables (218g)	78	30
Burger: hamburger: 1 large single patty, plain (137g)	62	26
Chilli con carne: (1 cup/253g)	25	25
Chow mein: (1 average serving/115g)	17	2

	RiskPoints ✗	LifePoints ✔
Corned beef: canned (1 slice/21g)	9	3
Corned beef: jellied loaf (2 slices/56g)	11	8
Cured dried beef: (28g)	3	7
Cured dried beef: thin-sliced (28g)	3	7
Curry: retail (1 average serving/115g)	26	6
Curry: retail, with rice (1 average serving/115g)	16	4
Dripping: (1 tbsp/13g)	47	0
Frankfurter: (1 frankfurter/57g)	51	7
Hotdog: in roll (1 link in roll/141g)	42	18
Hotdog: plain (1 link/98g)	38	13
Jerky: chopped and pressed (28g)	12	12
Kheema (1 average serving/115g)	112	21
Kofta: (1 average serving/115g)	79	23
Mince: extra lean, baked, medium (85g)	40	17
Mince: extra lean, grilled, medium (85g)	40	19
Mince: extra lean, pan-fried, medium (85g)	41	19
Mince: lean, baked, medium (85g)	45	17
Mince: lean, grilled, medium (85g)	46	19
Mince: lean, pan-fried, medium (85g)	47	19
Mince: regular, baked, medium (85g)	52	18
Mince: regular, grilled, medium (85g)	51	19

	RiskPoints ✗	LifePoints ✔
Mince: regular, pan-fried, medium (85g)	56	19
Pastrami: cured (2 slices/56g)	44	10
Porterhouse steak: lean and fat, grilled (85g)	56	19
Porterhouse steak: lean, grilled (85g)	27	21
Rib steak: lean and fat, grilled (85g)	65	18
Rump steak: lean and fat, grilled (85g)	26	20
Rump steak: lean, grilled (85g)	16	20
Sandwich: roast beef, plain (1 sandwich/139g)	34	23
Sandwich: roast beef, submarine style (1 submarine/216g)	53	28
Sandwich: roast beef, with cheese (1 sandwich/176g)	67	32
Sandwich: steak (1 sandwich/204g)	35	32
Sirloin steak: lean and fat, grilled (85g)	35	21
Sirloin steak: lean, grilled (85g)	17	23
Snack stick: smoked (1 stick/20g)	30	3
Soup: beef and noodles, canned (1 cup/8 fl. oz/244g)	17	5
Soup: beef and tomato with noodles (1 cup/8 fl. oz/244g)	23	5
Soup: beef and vegetable (1 cup/8 fl. oz/244g)	6	5
Soup: beef broth, bouillon and consommé (1 cup/8 fl. oz/241g)	0	2
Soup: oxtail (1 cup/8 fl. oz/253g)	9	2

	RiskPoints ✗	LifePoints ✔
Steak and kidney pie: (1 serving/250g)	166	25
Steak pudding: (1 average serving/115g)	52	11
Stew: beef, home-made (1 cup/252g)	13	22
Stroganoff: (1 serving/349g)	150	35
T-bone steak: lean and fat, grilled (85g)	54	19
T-bone steak: lean, grilled (85g)	26	21
Tenderloin: lean and fat, grilled (85g)	50	20
Tenderloin: lean and fat, roasted (85g)	64	18
Tenderloin: lean, grilled (85g)	23	22
Tenderloin: lean, roasted (85g)	27	20

Chicken

	RiskPoints ✗	LifePoints ✔
Breast: meat and skin, fried in batter (85g)	28	13
Breast: meat and skin, roasted (85g)	16	15
Breast: meat and skin, stewed (85g)	15	10
Breast: meat only, fried (85g)	10	17
Breast: meat only, roasted (85g)	7	15
Breast: meat only, stewed (85g)	6	11
Curry: with bone (1 average serving/115g)	36	14
Curry: without bone (1 average serving/115g)	48	18
Curry: without bone, retail (1 average serving/115g)	34	8

	RiskPoints ✗	LifePoints ✔
Curry: without bone, retail, with rice (1 average serving/115g)	19	5
Drumstick: meat and skin, fried in batter (1 drumstick/72g)	28	9
Drumstick: meat and skin, roasted (1 drumstick/52g)	14	7
Drumstick: meat and skin, stewed (1 drumstick/57g)	15	6
Drumstick: meat only, fried (1 drumstick/42g)	8	6
Drumstick: meat only, roasted (1 drumstick/44g)	6	6
Drumstick: meat only, stewed (1 drumstick/46g)	6	6
Fast food: boneless pieces, breaded and fried, plain (6 pieces/102g)	44	12
Fast food: boneless pieces, breaded and fried, with barbecue sauce (6 pieces/130g)	44	13
Fast food: boneless pieces, breaded and fried, with honey (6 pieces/115g)	43	12
Fast food: boneless pieces, breaded and fried, with mustard sauce (6 pieces/130g)	47	13
Fast food: boneless pieces, breaded and fried, with sweet and sour sauce (6 pieces/130g)	44	13
Fast food: breast or wing, light meat, breaded and fried (2 pieces/163g)	73	22
Fast food: drumstick or thigh, dark meat, breaded and fried (2 pieces/148g)	66	20

	RiskPoints ✗	LifePoints ✔
Fat: (1 tbsp/12g)	31	0
Frankfurter: (1 frankfurter/45g)	21	4
Giblets: fried (85g)	28	43
Giblets: simmered (85g)	10	32
Gizzard: simmered (½ cup/70g)	6	16
Heart: simmered (½ cup/70g)	13	25
Liver: simmered (½ cup/70g)	9	34
Meat: canned, boned, with stock (½ can/71g)	14	8
Meat and skin: fried in batter (85g)	36	11
Meat and skin: roasted (85g)	28	13
Meat and skin: stewed (85g)	26	10
Meat only: fried (85g)	19	15
Meat only: roasted (85g)	15	14
Meat only: stewed (85g)	14	11
Roll: light meat (1 slice/28g)	5	2
Salad: chicken and vegetable, with dressing (1 ½ cups/263g)	43	16
Salad: chicken and vegetable, without dressing (1 ½ cups/218g)	5	15
Salad spread: (1 tbsp/13g)	4	0
Sandwich: chicken fillet, plain (1 sandwich/182g)	73	19
Sandwich: chicken fillet, with cheese (1 sandwich/228g)	96	27
Soup: chicken and mushroom (1 cup/8 fl. oz/244g)	22	4
Soup: chicken and vegetables (1 cup/8 fl. oz/240g)	12	9

	RiskPoints ✗	LifePoints ✔
Soup: chicken noodle, canned, chunky, ready to serve (1 cup/8 fl. oz/240g)	15	9
Soup: cream of chicken (1 cup/8 fl. oz/248g)	34	9
Spread: canned (1 tbsp/13g)	3	1
Stock cube: dry (1 cube/5g)	0	0
Sweet and sour: (1 serving/453g)	41	25
Wing: meat and skin, fried in batter (1 wing/49g)	26	5
Wing: meat and skin, roasted (1 wing/34g)	16	4
Wing: meat and skin, stewed (1 wing/40g)	16	4
Wing: meat only, fried (1 wing/20g)	4	3
Wing: meat only, roasted (1 wing/21g)	4	3
Wing: meat only, stewed (1 wing/24g)	4	2

Duck

Meat and skin: roasted (85g)	61	11
Meat only: roasted (85g)	26	14

Game

Grouse: roasted, meat only (85g)	11	16
Hare: stewed, meat only (85g)	20	8
Partridge: roasted, meat only (85g)	15	8
Pheasant: roasted, meat only (85g)	19	11
Wild boar: roasted (85g)	9	8
Wild rabbit: stewed (85g)	7	9

Goose

	RiskPoints ✗	LifePoints ✔
Meat and skin: roasted (85g)	46	12
Meat only: roasted (85g)	29	15
Pâté de foie gras: goose liver pâté, smoked (28g)	31	11

Gravy

Au jus: (½ cup/119g)	0	3
Beef: (½ cup/116g)	10	3
Brown: dehydrated then prepared with water (½ cup/129g)	3	1
Chicken: (½ cup/119g)	16	2
Turkey: (½ cup/118g)	6	3

Lamb

Domestic: all cuts, lean and fat, cooked (85g)	56	20
Domestic: all cuts, lean only, cooked (85g)	21	21
Chop: lean and fat, grilled (85g)	80	19
Chop: lean and fat, roasted (85g)	81	18
Chop: lean only, grilled (85g)	29	21
Chop: lean only, roasted (85g)	30	19
Hotpot: (1 average serving/115g)	15	13
Irish stew: (1 average serving/115g)	30	7
Irish stew: weighed with bones (1 average serving/115g)	27	6
Kheema: (1 average serving/115g)	144	18
Leg: lean and fat, roasted (85g)	43	20

	RiskPoints ✘	LifePoints ✔
Leg: lean only, roasted (85g)	17	21
Moussaka: (1 serving/225g)	79	24
Mutton biriani: (1 average serving/115g)	83	10
Mutton curry: (1 average serving/115g)	168	19
Scotch broth: (1 cup/8 fl. oz/241g)	16	5
Shepherd's pie: (1 serving/225g)	42	21
New Zealand: all cuts, lean and fat, cooked (85g)	70	20
New Zealand: all cuts, lean only, cooked (85g)	24	22

Pork

	RiskPoints ✘	LifePoints ✔
Bacon: back, grilled (85g)	18	18
Bacon: gammon, grilled, pan-fried or roasted (85g)	111	22
Bacon: meatless (i.e. vegetarian, *see* "Legume & Bean Products" in the Legumes, Nuts & Seeds group.		
Bacon: streaky, grilled, pan-fried or roasted (85g)	81	24
Blade: lean and fat, braised (85g)	50	19
Blade: lean and fat, grilled (85g)	37	19
Blade: lean and fat, roasted (85g)	44	17
Blade: lean only, braised (85g)	35	20
Blade: lean only, grilled (85g)	28	20
Blade: lean only, roasted (85g)	33	23
Brains: braised (85g)	20	11
Chops: lean and fat, braised (85g)	37	15
Chops: lean and fat, grilled (85g)	36	20

	RiskPoints ✗	LifePoints ✔
Chops: lean and fat, pan-fried (85g)	40	17
Chops: lean and fat, roasted (85g)	37	17
Chops: lean only, braised (85g)	23	15
Chops: lean only, grilled (85g)	22	21
Chops: lean only, pan-fried (85g)	25	18
Chops: lean only, roasted (85g)	27	18
Ears: simmered (1 ear/111g)	32	5
Ham patty: grilled (1 patty/59g)	49	7
Ham: cured chopped, canned (1 slice/21g)	9	3
Ham: cured croquettes, grilled (1 croquette/59g)	49	7
Ham: cured, lean and fat, roasted (85g)	38	14
Ham: cured, lean only, roasted (85g)	11	17
Headcheese: pork (1 slice/28g)	11	3
Heart: braised (1 heart/129g)	16	38
Kidneys: braised (85g)	9	32
Lard: (1 tbsp/12g)	37	0
Leg: lean and fat, roasted (85g)	41	17
Leg: lean only, roasted (85g)	21	18
Sausage: fresh, cooked without additional fat (1 sausage/27g)	21	6
Liver: braised (85g)	9	45
Loin: lean and fat, braised (85g)	32	15
Loin: lean and fat, grilled (85g)	33	18
Loin: lean and fat, roasted (85g)	34	19
Loin: lean only, braised (85g)	21	16
Loin: lean only, grilled (85g)	23	19

	RiskPoints ✗	LifePoints ✔
Loin: lean only, roasted (85g)	22	20
Lungs: braised (85g)	6	20
Minced: cooked (85g)	49	16
Pork pie: (1 individual pie/210g)	121	34
Pork scratchings: (28g)	24	4
Sandwich: bacon (1 sandwich with 2 slices bacon/101g)	19	17
Sandwich: BLT (bacon, lettuce and tomato) (1 sandwich/151g)	34	15
Sandwich: ham and cheese (1 sandwich/146g)	48	20
Sandwich: ham, egg and cheese (1 sandwich/143g)	55	24
Sausage roll: (1 roll/55g)	58	2
Shoulder: lean and fat, roasted (85g)	50	16
Shoulder: lean only, roasted (85g)	30	18
Soup: ham and split pea, canned, chunky, ready to serve (1 cup/8 fl. oz/240g)	11	10
Spare ribs: lean and fat, braised (85g)	70	19
Tongue: braised (85g)	41	23
Trotters: pickled pig's feet (28g)	11	2

Rabbit

All cuts: roasted (85g)	17	21
All cuts: stewed (85g)	17	20

Sausages & luncheon meats

Beef luncheon meat: loaf (1 slice/28g)	23	7

	RiskPoints ✗	LifePoints ✔
Beef luncheon meat: thin-sliced (1 slice/4g)	0	1
Beef luncheon meat: cured, jellied (1 slice/28g)	2	9
Beerwurst: (beer salami) pork (1 slice/6g)	2	0
Beerwurst: (beer salami) pork (1 slice/23g)	22	3
Berliner: (1 slice/23g)	10	4
Blood sausage: or blood pudding (1 slice/25g)	25	3
Bockwurst: (1 link/65g)	49	9
Bologna: beef (1 slice/28g)	25	3
Bologna: beef and pork (1 slice/23g)	18	3
Bologna: pork (1 slice/23g)	11	3
Bratwurst: (1 link/85g)	59	13
Braunschweiger: (liver sausage) smoked (1 slice/18g)	14	12
Braunschweiger: cured pork (1 slice/18g)	14	12
Brotwurst: (1 link/70g)	52	12
Chicken liver pâté: canned (1 tbsp/13g)	4	9
Chorizo: (1 link/60g)	64	15
Cured ham: chopped, canned (1 slice/21g)	9	3
Cured ham: minced and pressed (1 slice/21g)	11	3
Goose liver pâté: see 'Pâté de foie gras' under Goose		
Ham and cheese spread: (1 tbsp/15g)	9	2
Ham luncheon meat: sliced (1 slice/28g)	7	5

	RiskPoints ✗	LifePoints ✔
Ham salad spread: (1 tbsp/15g)	5	1
Ham: chopped, not canned (1 slice/21g)	9	3
Ham: chopped, spiced, canned (1 slice/21g)	9	3
Headcheese: *see under* Pork		
Italian sausage: cooked (1 link/67g)	45	13
Liver cheese: cured pork (1 slice/38g)	25	22
Liver sausage: (liverwurst) pork (1 slice/18g)	14	11
Mixed pork and beef sausage: cooked (1 link/13g)	12	1
Mortadella: (1 slice/15g)	10	2
Pâté: de foie gras, canned, smoked (1 tbsp/13g)	14	6
Pâté: mixed meat or meat not specified (1 tbsp/13g)	9	3
Peppered loaf: (1 slice/28g)	4	5
Pepperoni: (1 slice/5g)	6	1
Pickle and pimiento loaf: made with pork (1 slice/28g)	16	4
Picnic loaf: (1 slice/28g)	12	4
Polish-style sausage: (1 sausage/227g)	175	33
Pork and beef: chopped together (1 slice/28g)	24	4
Pork and beef: sandwich spread (1 tbsp/15g)	6	1
Pork and olive loaf: (1 slice/28g)	12	4
Pork links: cooked (1 link/13g)	10	2
Pork luncheon meat: canned (1 slice/21g)	16	2

	RiskPoints ✗	LifePoints ✔
Sandwich: luncheon meat, submarine style (1 submarine/228g)	51	30
Sausage: meat, cooked (28g)	22	6
Sausage: luncheon type (1 slice/23g)	13	4
Sausage: smoked, linkpork (1 link/68g)	57	15
Sausage: smoked, linkpork, grilled (1 link/68g)	57	15
Thüringer: (1 slice/23g)	20	7
Turkey and ham: luncheon meat (1 slice/28g)	3	3
Vienna sausage: canned (1 sausage/16g)	11	1

Turkey

	RiskPoints ✗	LifePoints ✔
Boneless turkey meat: roasted (85g)	12	15
Breast: meat and skin, pre-basted and roasted (85g)	7	11
Breast: meat and skin, roasted (85g)	15	12
Dark meat: roasted (85g)	25	13
Giblets: simmered with some giblet fat (85g)	10	32
Leg: meat and skin, roasted (85g)	20	13
Light meat: roasted (85g)	6	13
Liver: simmered (85g)	12	35
Meat and skin: roasted (85g)	20	12
Meat only: roasted (85g)	10	13
Meat only: canned, with stock (85g)	14	11

	RiskPoints ✗	LifePoints ✔
Mince: cooked (1 patty/82g)	26	11
Patty: breaded, battered and fried (1 patty/85g)	42	9
Soup: turkey, canned, chunky, ready to serve (1 cup/8 fl. oz/236g)	11	16
Thigh: meat and skin, pre-basted and roasted (85g)	18	10
Turkey roll: made from light and dark meat (85g)	14	10
Turkey sticks: breaded, battered and fried (1 stick/64g)	27	6
Wing: meat and skin, roasted (1 wing/186g)	57	26

Veal

	RiskPoints ✗	LifePoints ✔
Lean and fat meat: braised (85g)	24	20
Lean and fat meat: breaded and pan-fried (85g)	19	19
Lean and fat meat: pan-fried, not breaded (85g)	20	21
Lean and fat meat: roasted (85g)	17	17
Lean only: braised (85g)	18	20
Lean only: breaded and pan-fried (85g)	13	20
Lean only, pan-fried, not breaded (85g)	9	22
Lean only: roasted (85g)	12	18
Mince: grilled (85g)	19	17

Venison

	RiskPoints ✗	LifePoints ✔
Roasted (85g)	7	14

FISH & SEAFOOD

NOTE: throughout this section, 'moist heat' includes cooking methods such as steaming, stewing and inclusion in soups and sauces; 'dry heat' includes methods such as grilling and baking.

	RiskPoints ✗	LifePoints ✔
Abalone: fried (85g)	14	10
Anchovy: canned in oil, drained solids (5 anchovies/20g)	4	5
Bass: freshwater, cooked dry heat (1 fillet/62g)	7	11
Bass: *see also* 'Sea bass'		
Bass: striped, cooked dry heat (1 fillet/124g)	9	18
Burbot: cooked dry heat (1 fillet/90g)	2	14
Carp: cooked dry heat (1 fillet/170g)	30	25
Catfish: breaded and fried (1 fillet/87g)	28	13
Caviar: black and red granular (1 tbsp/16g)	7	11
Clam: breaded and fried (10 small clams/94g)	26	22
Clam: canned, drained solids (85g)	4	27
Clam: canned, with liquid (85g)	0	8
Clam: cooked moist heat (10 small clams/94g)	4	28
Cod liver oil: (1 tbsp/13g)	34	0
Cod: canned, solids and liquid (1 can/312g)	6	30
Cod: cooked dry heat (1 fillet/180g)	3	22
Cod: dried and salted (85g)	5	29

	RiskPoints ✗	LifePoints ✔
Crab: blue, cake (1 cake/60g)	11	15
Crab: blue, canned (85g)	2	11
Crab: blue, cooked moist heat (85g)	3	19
Crayfish: wild, cooked moist heat (85g)	2	14
Croaker: breaded and fried (1 fillet/87g)	27	15
Cuttlefish: cooked moist heat (85g)	2	31
Eel: cooked dry heat (1 fillet/159g)	59	24
Fish and chips: 1 fillet of plaice fried in batter and 1 regular order of chips fried in vegetable oil (256g)	111	19
Fish fillet: battered or breaded and fried (1 fillet/91g)	27	12
Fish fingers (1 finger/28g)	8	4
Fish pie: (1 serving/200g)	36	17
Flatfish: (flounder and sole species) cooked dry heat (1 fillet/127g)	4	18
Gefilte fish: sweet recipe (1 piece/42g)	1	3
Grouper: cooked dry heat (1 fillet/202g)	6	21
Haddock: cooked dry heat (1 fillet/150g)	3	23
Haddock: smoked (85g)	2	14
Halibut: Atlantic, cooked dry heat (½ fillet/159g)	11	28
Halibut: Greenland, cooked dry heat (½ fillet/159g)	70	18

	RiskPoints ✗	LifePoints ✔
Herring: Atlantic, cooked dry heat (1 fillet/143g)	41	25
Herring: Atlantic, kippered (1 fillet/40g)	12	13
Herring: Atlantic, pickled (1 piece/15g)	6	3
Kedgeree: (1 serving/115g)	20	14
Kipper: see 'Herring'		
Ling: cooked dry heat (1 fillet/151g)	3	20
Lobster: cooked moist heat (85g)	1	14
Lox: see 'Salmon'		
Mackerel: Atlantic, cooked dry heat (1 fillet/88g)	39	20
Mackerel: canned, drained solids (1 can/190g)	29	33
Mackerel: king, cooked dry heat (1 fillet/308g)	19	48
Monkfish: cooked dry heat (85g)	4	9
Mullet: cooked dry heat (1 fillet/93g)	11	12
Mussels: cooked moist heat (85g)	9	24
Ocean perch: Atlantic, cooked dry heat (1 fillet/50g)	2	7
Oyster: breaded and fried (6 medium/88g)	27	23
Oyster: canned (85g)	5	22
Oyster: stew, canned, condensed (1 cup/8 fl. oz/246g)	37	18
Oyster: wild, cooked moist heat (6 medium/42g)	5	21
Perch: cooked dry heat (1 fillet/46g)	1	8

	RiskPoints ✘	LifePoints ✔
Pike: cooked dry heat (1 fillet/124g)	4	23
Pike: northern, cooked dry heat (½ fillet/155g)	3	22
Pollack: Atlantic, cooked dry heat (½ fillet/151g)	4	23
Roe: cooked dry heat (85g)	17	25
Salad: seafood, vegetable and pasta, without dressing (1½ cups/417g)	52	24
Salad: tuna (85g)	19	11
Salmon: Atlantic, wild, cooked dry heat (½ fillet/154g)	31	39
Salmon: canned, drained solids with bone (85g)	15	11
Salmon: chum, cooked dry heat (½ fillet/154g)	18	28
Salmon: cooked dry heat (½ fillet/155g)	42	26
Salmon: pink, canned, solids with bone and liquid (85g)	12	18
Salmon: pink, cooked dry heat (½ fillet/124g)	13	23
Salmon: smoked (85g)	9	14
Salmon: smoked (lox), regular (85g)	9	14
Sandwich: tuna salad, submarine style (1 submarine/256g)	69	29
Sardine: Atlantic, canned in oil, drained solids with bone (2 sardines/24g)	6	11
Sardine: Atlantic, canned in oil, drained solids with bone (1 can/92g)	26	22

	RiskPoints ✗	LifePoints ✔
Sardine: Pacific, canned in tomato sauce, drained solids with bone (2 sardines/76g)	22	17
Sardine: Pacific, canned in tomato sauce, drained solids with bone (1 can/370g)	110	51
Scallop: breaded and fried (2 large scallops/31g)	8	3
Scampi: breaded and fried (6 pieces/164g)	62	16
Sea bass: cooked dry heat (1 fillet/101g)	6	10
Sea trout: cooked dry heat (1 fillet/186g)	21	25
Shad: cooked dry heat (1 fillet/144g)	63	24
Shark: batter-dipped and fried (85g)	29	11
Prawn: breaded and fried (4 large shrimp/30g)	9	5
Prawn: canned (85g)	4	11
Prawn: cooked moist heat (4 large shrimp/22g)	0	3
Prawn: salad sandwich with mayonnaise (1 sandwich/148g)	29	16
Smelt: cooked dry heat (85g)	6	15
Snapper: cooked dry heat (1 fillet/170g)	7	21
Sole: see 'Flatfish'		
Spiny lobster: cooked moist heat (1 lobster/163g)	7	30
Squid: fried (85g)	15	12
Sturgeon: cooked dry heat (85g)	11	18

	RiskPoints ✗	LifePoints ✔
Sturgeon: smoked (85g)	9	20
Swordfish: cooked dry heat (85g)	10	18
Trout: cooked dry heat (1 fillet/62g)	13	17
Trout: rainbow, cooked dry heat (1 fillet/71g)	12	17
Tuna: canned in oil, drained solids (1 can/171g)	35	28
Tuna: canned in oil, drained solids (85g)	17	19
Tuna: canned in water, drained solids (1 can/165g)	3	28
Tuna: canned in water, drained solids (85g)	1	20
Turbot: cooked dry heat (½ fillet/159g)	15	20
Whelk: cooked moist heat (85g)	1	26
Whitefish: cooked dry heat (1 fillet/154g)	28	23
Whitefish: smoked (85g)	1	15
Whiting: cooked dry heat (1 fillet/72g)	3	13

DAIRY
Butter

Butter: (1 pat/5g)	18	0
Ghee: anhydrous butter oil (1 tbsp/13g)	46	0

Cheese

Brie: (28g)	36	5
Camembert: (28g)	32	5
Cheddar: (28g)	42	5

	RiskPoints ✗	LifePoints ✔
Cheese fondue: (1 serving/80g)	77	12
Cheese soufflé: (1 cup/136g)	86	16
Cheshire: (28g)	40	5
Cottage: creamed, large or small curd (28g)	5	2
Cottage: creamed, large or small curd (113g)	24	8
Cottage: lowfat 2% fat (28g)	2	2
Cottage: lowfat 2% fat (113g)	10	9
Cream cheese: (28g)	46	1
Edam: (28g)	36	6
Feta: (28g)	31	7
Fontina: (28g)	40	7
Gjetost: (28g)	40	7
Goat: hard type (28g)	52	7
Goat: semi-soft type (28g)	43	3
Goat: soft type (28g)	30	3
Gouda: (28g)	36	6
Gruyère: (28g)	39	7
Mozzarella: part skimmed milk (28g)	21	4
Mozzarella: whole milk (28g)	27	3
Neufchâtel: (28g)	31	1
Parmesan: grated (28g)	40	8
Parmesan: grated (1 tbsp/5g)	7	1
Parmesan: solid (28g)	34	7
Port Salut: (28g)	35	5
Processed: (28g)	32	5
Provolone: (28g)	35	6

	RiskPoints ✗	LifePoints ✔
Ricotta: part skimmed milk (¼ cup/62g)	22	5
Ricotta: whole milk (¼ cup/62g)	38	5
Romano: (28g)	35	6
Roquefort: (28g)	40	5
Sandwich: cheese and pickle, made with cheddar (1 sandwich/105g)	53	15
Sandwich: cheese and tomato, made with cheddar (1 sandwich/150g)	53	17
Swiss: (28g)	37	7
Swiss: pasteurized, processed (28g)	32	6
Tilsit: whole milk (28g)	35	6
Welsh rarebit (1 serving/60g)	62	8

Cream

	RiskPoints ✗	LifePoints ✔
Dessert topping: non-dairy, powdered (amount to make 1 tbsp/1g)	3	0
Dessert topping: non-dairy, pressurized (1 tbsp/4g)	5	0
Double: (1 tbsp/15g)	17	0
Single: (1 tbsp/15g)	13	0
Sour cream: (1 tbsp/12g)	11	0
Substitute: non-dairy powder (1 tsp/2g)	4	0
Whipped cream topping: pressurized (1 tbsp/3g)	3	0
Whipping cream: heavy (1 tbsp/15g)	25	0
Whipping cream: light (1 tbsp/15g)	21	0

Eggs: Chicken

	RiskPoints ✘	LifePoints ✔
Dried: (1 tbsp/5g)	5	3
Dried: white only, powder (¼ cup sifted/27g)	0	9
Dried: yolk only (1 tbsp/4g)	6	2
Egg custard: baked (½ cup/141g)	24	8
Egg substitute: powder (1 tsp/0.9g)	3	4
Fried: (1 large egg/46g)	17	6
Hard-boiled: (1 large egg/50g)	13	7
Omelette: (1 large egg/59g)	16	6
Omelette: (2 eggs/120g)	34	12
Poached: (1 large egg/50g)	12	6
Quiche lorraine: (1 serving/115g)	107	15
Raw: yolk and white (1 large egg/50g)	12	7
Raw: white only (1 large egg white/33g)	0	1
Raw: yolk only (1 large egg yolk/16g)	12	5
Sandwich: egg and cheese (1 sandwich/146g)	49	20
Sandwich: egg mayonnaise (1 sandwich/135g)	48	15
Sandwich: egg, cress and mayonnaise (1 sandwich/145g)	36	17
Scotch egg: (1 egg/115g)	67	13
Scrambled: (1 egg/60g)	18	7

Eggs: Duck

Raw: (1 egg/70g)	24	17

Eggs: Goose

	RiskPoints ✗	LifePoints ✔
Raw: (1 egg/144g)	47	27

Eggs: Quail

Raw: (1 egg/9g)	2	1

Milk: Cow's

Buttermilk: cultured from skimmed milk (1 cup/245g)	10	10
Buttermilk: dried (1 tbsp/6g)	1	3
Condensed: canned, sweetened (1 fl. oz/38g)	15	3
Dried: Skimmed milk non-fat solids (¼ cup/30g)	1	15
Dried: whole milk (¼ cup/32g)	40	12
Evaporated: canned, unsweetened (1 fl. oz/31g)	10	2
Malted milk beverage: (1 cup milk + 3 tsp powder/265g)	44	17
Malted milk beverage: dry powder (3 tsp/21g)	6	5
Malted milk beverage: dry powder, chocolate (3 tsp/21g)	3	2
Milkshake: thick chocolate (1 container/300g)	37	16
Milkshake: thick vanilla (1 container/313g)	44	19
Whole: (1 cup/244g)	41	12
Semi-skimmed: (1 cup/244g)	22	14
Skimmed milk: (1 cup 245g)	2	12

Milk: Goat's

	RiskPoints ✗	LifePoints ✔
Goat's milk: (1 cup/244g)	48	9

Milk: Sheep's

Ewe's milk: (1 cup/245g)	84	22

Yogurt

Low-fat: (½ container/113g)	8	8
Low-fat: with fruit (½ container/113g)	5	7
Skimmed milk: (½ container/113g)	0	9
Whole milk: (½ container/113g)	17	5

Drinks

Fruit juices are listed in Food Group One. Vegetable juices are listed in Food Group Two. Alcoholic drinks are generally double-zero foods, but see 'What about alcohol?' on page 50.

	RiskPoints ✗	LifePoints ✔
Cappuccino: (coffee made with full-fat milk and chocolate) (1 cup/212g)	33	1
Carbonated soft drink: (e.g. lemonade) (12 fl. oz can/368g)	0	0
Cocoa: home-made from hot milk (1 cup/8 fl. oz/250g)	42	14
Coffee: brewed (6 fl. oz/177g)	0	0
Coffee: instant, decaffeinated (1 rounded tsp/2g)	0	0
Coffee: instant, caffeinated (1 rounded tsp/2g)	0	0
Coffee substitute: cereal grain beverage powder (1 tsp/2g)	0	0
Cola: (12 fl. oz can/355g)	0	0
Cola: low-calorie (12 fl. oz can/355g)	0	0
Eggnog: (½ cup/4 fl. oz/127g)	42	7
Ginger ale: (12 fl. oz can/366g)	0	0
Lemonade: see 'Carbonated soft drink'		
Malted milk: with added nutrients, prepared with milk (1 cup/8 fl. oz milk plus 3 heaped tsp/265g)	40	34
Malted milk: with no added nutrients, prepared with milk (1 cup/8 fl. oz milk plus 3 heaped tsp/265g)	44	17

	RiskPoints ✗	LifePoints ✔
Milkshake: chocolate (10 fl. oz/283g)	49	16
Milkshake: vanilla (10 fl. oz/283g)	39	14
Tea: herb (6 fl. oz/178g)	0	0
Tea: no milk or sugar (6 fl. oz/178g)	0	0
Tea: with milk, no sugar (1 cup/8 fl. oz/238g)	12	3
Tea: with milk, one sugar (1 cup/8 fl. oz/242g)	12	3
Tea: with milk, two sugars (1 cup/8 fl. oz/246g)	12	3
Tonic water: (12 fl. oz can/366g)	0	0
Vinegar: cider (1 tbsp/15g)	0	0
Water: bottled e.g. Perrier (1 cup/8 fl. oz/237g)	0	0

Biscuits & Cookies

Animal crackers: (10 crackers/25g)	8	2
Brandy snap: (1 snap/15g)	7	0
Brownie: chocolate, California Cake & Cookie, 98% fat-free (one slice/29g)	2	5
Brownie: (commercial) (1 large brownie/56g)	22	4
Brownie: home-made (1 brownie/33g)	24	2
Brownie: regular, prepared from dry mix (1 brownie/33g)	16	1
Chocolate biscuit: fully coated (1 biscuit/15g)	10	0

	RiskPoints ✗	LifePoints ✔
Chocolate chip cookie: (commercial) soft type (1 cookie/15g)	9	0
Chocolate chip cookie: home-made, with butter (1 cookie/15g)	15	1
Chocolate chip cookie: home-made, with margarine (1 cookie/15g)	10	1
Chocolate chip cookie: made from dry mix (1 cookie/15g)	9	1
Chocolate cookie: sandwich with creme filling, regular (1 cookie/15g)	7	1
Chocolate cookie: sandwich with creme filling, regular chocolate-coated (1 cookie/17g)	11	1
Coconut: home-made (1 cookie/24g)	20	0
Custard cream: (1 biscuit/14g)	15	0
Digestive biscuit: Asda Healthy Choice (25% less fat) (1 biscuit/15g)	7	1
Digestive biscuit: chocolate (1 biscuit/15g)	13	0
Digestive biscuit: chocolate, Asda Healthy Choice (25% less fat) (1 biscuit/13g)	8	0
Digestive biscuit: plain (1 biscuit/15g)	9	1
Fig bar: (1 cookie/16g)	2	1
Flapjack: (1 flapjack/33g)	21	2
Fortune cookie: (1 cookie/8g)	0	0
Gingerbread: (1 biscuit/33g)	10	1

	RiskPoints ✗	LifePoints ✔
Gingernut biscuit: home-made (1 biscuit/15g)	7	0
Gingernut biscuit: retail (1 biscuit/15g)	5	1
Ladyfinger: with lemon juice and rind (1 ladyfinger/11g)	2	1
Oatmeal cookie: (commercial) soft type (1 cookie/15g)	5	1
Oatmeal cookie: home-made, with raisins (1 cookie/15g)	6	1
Oatmeal cookie: made from dry mix (1 cookie/15g)	7	1
Peanut butter cookie: (commercial) soft type (1 cookie/15g)	9	0
Peanut butter cookie: home-made (1 cookie/15g)	8	1
Raisin cookie: soft type (1 cookie/15g)	5	1
Rich tea biscuit: Asda Healthy Choice (25% less fat) (1 biscuit/10g)	3	0
Shortbread: (1 cookie/15g)	9	0
Shortbread: home-made, with butter (1 cookie/15g)	23	1
Shortbread: home-made, with margarine (1 cookie/15g)	12	1
Wafer biscuit: filled (1 biscuit/14g)	10	0

Cakes, Pastries & Puddings

	RiskPoints ✗	LifePoints ✔
Angelfood cake: (1 serving/53g)	0	2
Apple crumble: (1 serving/115g)	21	3
Apple pie: (1 serving/155g)	48	5

	RiskPoints ✗	LifePoints ✔
Apple strudel: (1 slice/71g)	19	2
Bath bun see 'Chelsea bun'		
Battenburg cake: (1 slice/30g)	13	2
Bread and butter pudding: (1 serving/115g)	34	6
Carrot cake: California Cake & Cookie, 98% fat-free (1 slice/29g)	2	1
Carrot cake: regular full-fat, with cream cheese icing (1 serving/111g)	73	6
Carrot cake: without icing (1 serving/70g)	27	7
Cheesecake: (1 serving/80g)	69	4
Chelsea bun: (1 bun/30g)	10	2
Cherry pie: (1 serving/125g)	34	2
Chocolate cake: with chocolate icing (1 serving/64g)	26	3
Christmas pudding: (1 serving/115g)	46	6
Coffeen cake: creme-filled, with chocolate icing (1 serving/90g)	24	5
Cream horn: (1 horn/45g)	56	1
Cream puff: (1 cream puff shell/66g)	42	6
Custard tart: individual (1 tart/30g)	12	1
Danish pastry: (1 pastry/65g)	36	7
Doughnut: creme filling (1 doughnut/85g)	52	7
Doughnut: jam filling (1 doughnut/85g)	39	6
Doughnut: ring, glazed (1 medium doughnut/60g)	34	6

	RiskPoints ✗	LifePoints ✔
Doughnut: ring, plain (1 medium doughnut/47g)	26	3
Eccles cake: (1 cake/45g)	34	2
Eclair: custard-filled, with chocolate glaze (1 eclair/100g)	39	7
Fancy iced cakes: individual (1 cake/45g)	31	1
Fruit spice cake: California Cake & Cookie, 98% fat-free (one slice/28g)	0	2
Fruitcake: (1 small serving/43g)	9	1
Gateau: (1 slice/60g)	42	5
Gingerbread cake: (1 serving/74g)	30	5
Ice cream cone: cake or wafer type (1 cone/4g)	0	0
Icing: chocolate, made with butter (1 serving/50g)	26	0
Icing: chocolate, made with margarine (1 serving/50g)	14	0
Icing: glaze (1 serving/27g)	5	0
Icing: vanilla, made with butter (1 serving/48g)	9	0
Icing: vanilla, made with margarine (1 serving/48g)	12	0
Instant dessert: made up with semi-skimmed milk (1 serving/75g)	20	3
Instant dessert: made up with skimmed milk (1 serving/75g)	16	3
Instant dessert: made up with whole milk (1 serving/75g)	27	3
Jam tart: (1 tart/40g)	17	1
Jelly: made with semi-skimmed milk (1 serving/75g)	2	2

	RiskPoints ✗	LifePoints ✔
Jelly: made with skimmed milk (1 serving/75g)	0	2
Jelly: made with water (1 serving/75g)	0	0
Jelly: made with whole milk (1 serving/75g)	6	1
Lemon curd: (1 tbsp/20g)	10	0
Lemon meringue pie: (1 serving/113g)	24	5
Madeira cake: (1 serving/74g)	48	2
Marble cake: no icing (1 serving/73g)	31	3
Marzipan: (commercial) (1 oz/28g)	0	0
Marzipan: home-made (1 oz/28g)	0	0
Meringue: (1 meringue 10g)	0	0
Meringue: with cream (1 meringue/30g)	33	1
Milk pudding: (e.g. sago, rice, semolina, tapioca) made with semi-skimmed milk (1 average serving/115g)	9	6
Milk pudding: (e.g. sago, rice, semolina, tapioca) made with skimmed milk (1 average serving/115g)	0	4
Milk pudding: (e.g. sago, rice, semolina, tapioca) made with whole milk (1 average serving/115g)	23	4
Mince pie: (1 individual pie/50g)	29	2
Mousse: chocolate (1 average serving/115g)	15	6
Mousse: chocolate, rich (1 average serving/115g)	19	0
Mousse: frozen (1 average serving/115g)	31	5

	RiskPoints ✘	LifePoints ✔
Mousse: fruit (1 average serving/115g)	16	6
Pecan pie: (1 serving/122g)	67	8
Pie crust: short-crust, baked (1 serving/23g)	19	2
Pineapple upside-down cake: (1 serving/115g)	34	7
Pound cake: made with butter (1 serving/53g)	57	4
Puff pastry: baked (1 oz/28g)	27	2
Pumpkin pie: (1 serving/155g)	36	9
Rice pudding: canned (1 can/5 oz/142g)	26	4
Sponge cake: (1 serving/38g)	2	3
Sponge cake: fatless (1 slice/30g)	4	3
Sponge pudding: home-made (1 serving/75g)	30	4
Suet pudding: (1 serving/115g)	87	5
Swiss roll: chocolate, individual (1 roll/50g)	14	2
Treacle tart: (1 serving/115g)	47	4
Trifle: (1 serving/115g)	24	4
Yellow cake: with chocolate icing (1 serving/64g)	27	3

Dressings & Sauces

Barbecue sauce: (½ cup/4 fl. oz/125g)	5	3
Barbecue sauce: home-made, (½ cup/125g) made with butter	122	7
Bolognese sauce (¾ cup/6 fl. oz/200g)	54	21
Brown sauce: hot (1 tbsp/15g)	0	0

	RiskPoints ✘	LifePoints ✔
Brown sauce: sweet (1 tbsp/15g)	0	0
Casserole sauce: dry mix, made up (½ cup/115g)	1	0
Cheese sauce: made with milk (½ cup/4 fl. oz/140g)	35	9
Chilli pickle: oily (1 tbsp/15g)	9	1
Chilli sauce: (1 tbsp/15g)	0	0
Chocolate nut spread: (1 tbsp/15g)	12	0
Chocolate spread: (1 tbsp/15g)	14	0
Cranberry sauce: (½ cup/115g)	0	0
Curry paste: (1 tbsp/15g)	7	1
Curry sauce: canned (½ cup/115g)	14	1
Curry sauce: onion, made with butter (½ cup/130g)	156	5
Curry sauce: onion, made with vegetable oil (½ cup/130g)	97	4
Curry sauce: sweet (½ cup/130g)	18	3
Curry sauce: tomato and onion (½ cup/130g)	62	4
Fruit spread: (1 tbsp/15g)	0	0
Hollandaise sauce: prepared with vegetable oil, dehydrated, and then made with milk and butter (1 cup/8 fl. oz/254g)	313	9
Horseradish sauce: (1 tbsp/15g)	3	0
Hot pepper sauce: (1 tbsp/15g)	0	0
Ice cream sauce: topping (1 tbsp/15g)	0	0
Jaggery: (1 average serving/30g)	0	0
Ketchup: (1 tbsp/15g)	2	0
Lime pickle: oily (1 tbsp/15g)	5	1

	RiskPoints ✗	LifePoints ✔
Mango chutney: oily (1 tbsp/15g)	4	0
Mango chutney: sweet (1 tbsp/15g)	0	0
Mango pickle: oily (1 tbsp/15g)	5	1
Mayonnaise: home-made (1 tbsp/13g)	25	0
Mayonnaise: retail (1 tbsp/13g)	24	0
Mayonnaise: retail, reduced calorie (1 tbsp/13g)	9	0
Mayonnaise: made with soya bean oil (1 tbsp/13g)	27	0
Mayonnaise: made with soybean and safflower oil (1 tbsp/13g)	27	0
Mayonnaise: made without dairy products (i.e. vegan) (1 tbsp/14g)	16	0
Mint sauce: (1 tbsp/15g)	0	0
Mint sauce: homemade (1 tbsp/15g)	0	0
Mixed vegetable pickle (1 tbsp/15g)	0	0
Mornay sauce (½ cup/168g)	64	15
Mustard: smooth (1 tbsp/15g)	3	0
Mustard: wholegrain (1 tbsp/15g)	3	0
Mustard: plain (1 tbsp/17g)	6	2
Mustard: prepared with cream (1 tbsp/17g)	9	0
Onion sauce: made with semi-skimmed milk (½ cup/125g)	16	6
Onion sauce: made with skimmed milk (½ cup/125g)	12	6
Onion sauce: made with whole milk (½ cup/125g)	26	6
Pasta sauce: tomato-based (½ cup/130g)	4	6

	RiskPoints ✘	LifePoints ✔
Pasta sauce: white (½ cup/130g)	66	11
Pesto sauce (1 tbsp/15g)	17	2
Piccalilli (1 tbsp/15g)	0	0
Pickle: sweet (1 tbsp/15g)	2	0
Raita: plain (½ cup/ 113g)	81	5
Raita: yogurt and gram flour (½ cup/ 113g)	35	5
Redcurrant jelly (1 tbsp/15g)	0	0
Relish: corn, cucumber or onion (1 tbsp/25g)	0	0
Sage and onion stuffing: home-made (½ cup/125g)	46	7
Salad cream (1 tbsp/13g)	10	0
Salad cream: reduced-calorie (1 tbsp/13g)	5	0
Salad dressing: fat-free (1 tbsp/15g)	0	0
Salad dressing: French, home-made (1 tbsp/15g)	27	0
Salad dressing: low-fat (1 tbsp/15g)	1	0
Salad dressing: oil and lemon (1 tbsp/15g)	26	0
Salad dressing: yogurt-based (1 tbsp/15g)	10	0
Salad dressing: yogurt-based, home-made (1 tbsp/15g)	1	1
Salad dressing: blue and Roquefort cheese (1 tbsp/15g)	20	0
Salad dressing: French (1 tbsp/14g)	24	0
Salad dressing: French, low-fat (1 tbsp/16g)	2	0

	RiskPoints ✗	LifePoints ✔
Salad dressing: Italian, low-fat (1 tbsp/15g)	3	0
Salad dressing: thousand island (1 tbsp/15g)	13	0
Salad dressing: thousand island, low-fat (1 tbsp/15g)	4	0
Salad dressing: vinegar and oil (1 tbsp/15g)	19	0
Sandwich spread (1 tbsp/15g)	3	0
Sauces from dry mix (e.g. parsley onion and bread) made up (½ cup/130g)	13	3
Sesame seed dressing (1 tbsp/15g)	17	0
Stuffing mix: made up (½ cup/125g)	7	9
Sweet and sour sauce (½ cup/4 fl oz/156g)	0	2
Sweet and sour sauce: canned (½ cup/130g)	0	1
Sweet and sour sauce: takeaway (½ cup/130g)	11	5
Tartar sauce (1 tbsp/20g)	12	0
Teriyaki sauce (1 tbsp/18g)	0	0
Tomato and mushroom sauce (½ cup/130g)	11	4
Tomato base sauce: home-made (½ cup/130g)	16	4
Tomato base sauce: retail (½ cup/130g)	16	4
Tzatziki (½ cup/160g)	34	6
White sauce: made with semi-skimmed milk (½ cup/130g)	28	8
White sauce: made with skimmed milk (½ cup/130g)	20	8

	RiskPoints ✗	LifePoints ✔
White sauce: made with whole milk (½ cup/130g)	42	7
White sauce: packet mix, made up with semi-skimmed milk (½ cup/130g)	7	7
White sauce: packet mix, made up with skimmed milk (½ cup/130g)	2	7
White sauce: packet mix, made up with whole milk (½ cup/130g)	15	7
Worcestershire sauce (1 tbsp/15g)	0	1

Snacks & Sweets

	RiskPoints ✗	LifePoints ✔
Banana chips (1 oz/28g)	61	1
Boiled sweets (standard 1 oz serving/28g)	0	0
Bombay mix (1 oz/28g)	23	4
Butterscotch or caramel topping (2 tbsp/41g)	0	0
Caramel cookie bar (1 pkt/57g)	33	3
Carob cookie (1 bar/3 oz/87g)	71	17
Cereal and potato flour snacks (1 packet/25g)	14	1
Cereal chewy bar (1 bar/24g)	9	1
Cereal crunchy bar (1 bar/24g)	13	2
Cherries: glacé (10 fruit/68g)	0	0
Chewing gum (1 stick/3g)	0	0
Chewy sweets (standard 1 oz serving/28g)	6	0
Chocolate: after dinner mints (2 pieces/8g)	4	0
Chocolate: diabetic (standard 1 oz serving/28g)	38	2

	RiskPoints ✗	LifePoints ✔
Chocolate: fancy and filled (standard 1 oz serving/28g)	24	1
Chocolate: white (standard 1 oz serving/28g)	39	2
Chocolate: baking chocolate, unsweetened (1 square/1 oz/28g)	69	3
Chocolate: caramels in milk chocolate (1 pkt/55g)	29	4
Chocolate: fudge (1 piece/17g)	6	0
Chocolate: milk (1 bar/44g)	60	4
Chocolate: milk chocolate coated peanuts (10 pieces/40g)	43	5
Chocolate: milk chocolate coated raisins (10 pieces/10g)	6	0
Chocolate: semi-sweet chocolate, made with butter (1 oz/28g)	37	1
Chocolate: semi-sweet chocolate, regular (1 oz/28g)	37	1
Chocolate: snack bar (1 bar/2.1 oz/60g)	35	4
Chocolate: sweet chocolate (1 oz/28g)	42	1
Chocolate: wafer bar (1 bar/1.6 oz/46g)	57	4
Chocolate covered bar: with fruit/ nuts and wafer biscuit (standard 1 oz serving/28g)	28	2
Chocolate covered caramels (standard 1 oz serving/28g)	22	2
Coconut ice (standard 1 oz serving/28g)	22	2
Corn and starch snacks (1 pkt/25g)	25	1
Corn-based packet snacks (1 pkt/25g)	22	2

	RiskPoints ✗	LifePoints ✔
Fruit leather bar (1 bar/23g)	6	0
Fruit pastilles (standard 1 oz serving/28g)	0	0
Fudge (standard 1 oz serving/28g)	19	1
Halva: (Greek) (standard 1 oz serving/28g)	22	3
Halva: carrot (standard 1 oz serving/28g)	23	2
Halva: semolina (standard 1 oz serving/28g)	20	0
Halwa: (Asian) (standard 1 oz serving/28g)	9	0
Honey: strained or extracted (1 tbsp/21g)	0	0
Honeycomb (standard 1 oz serving/28g)	3	0
Ice cream: chocolate (1 serving/66g)	40	4
Ice cream: strawberry (1 serving/66g)	13	3
Ice cream: vanilla, regular (1 serving/66g)	40	3
Ice cream: vanilla, rich (1 serving/74g)	55	3
Ice cream: vanilla, soft-serve (1 serving/86g)	48	5
Ice cream: yogurt, soft-serve (1 serving/72g)	18	4
Ice cream bar: chocolate covered (1 bar/74g)	83	4
Instant soup powder: as served (1 cup/240g)	13	1
Instant soup powder: calorie-controlled, as served (1 cup/240g)	9	4

	RiskPoints ✗	LifePoints ✔
Jam: diabetic (1 tbsp/20g)	0	0
Jam: fruit with edible seeds (1 tbsp/20g)	0	0
Jam: reduced sugar (1 tbsp/20g)	0	0
Jam: stone fruit (1 tbsp/20g)	0	0
Jams and preserves: others (1 tbsp/20g)	0	0
Jellies (1 packet/14g)	4	0
Jellybeans (10 small/11g)	5	0
Lemon curd: home-made (1 tbsp/20g)	14	1
Liquorice shapes (standard 1 oz serving/28g)	0	5
Maize and rice flour snacks (1 packet/25g)	13	2
Marmalade: diabetic (1 tbsp/20g)	0	0
Marmalade: orange (1 tbsp/20g)	5	0
Marshmallows (1 regular/7g)	2	0
Mincemeat (standard 1 oz serving/28g)	3	0
Mincemeat: vegetarian (standard 1 oz serving/28g)	8	0
Molasses: blackstrap (1 tbsp/20g)	0	5
Molasses: regular (1 tbsp/20g)	2	1
Muesli bar (1 bar/24g)	12	2
Nougat (standard 1 oz serving/28g)	6	1
Nuts and raisins (1 oz /28g)	23	5
Oriental mix (standard 1 oz serving/28g)	28	6
Peanut bar (1 bar/45g)	37	6
Peanut brittle (1 oz /28g)	13	3

	RiskPoints ✗	LifePoints ✔
Peanuts and raisins (1 oz/28g)	18	6
Peppermint creams (standard 1 oz serving/28g)	0	0
Peppermints (standard 1 oz serving/28g)	0	0
Popcorn: air-popped (1 cup/8g)	0	1
Popcorn: caramel-coated (1 cup/35g)	11	1
Popcorn: cheese flavour (1 cup/11g)	9	1
Popcorn: oil-popped (1 cup/11g)	7	1
Pot savouries: instant noodles, rice or chilli, made up (1 average serving/115g)	8	2
Potato sticks (1 oz/28g)	24	3
Pretzels: hard, salted (10 twists/60g)	5	11
Sesame bar: brittle type (1 oz/28g)	23	7
Sherbet sweets (standard 1 oz serving/28g)	0	0
Sorbet ice: made with water and fruit only (1 serving/96g)	0	0
Sugar: Demerara (1 tsp/4g)	0	0
Sugar: brown (1 tsp/4g)	0	0
Sugar: granulated (1 tsp/4g)	0	0
Sugar: icing (1 tbsp unsifted/8g)	0	0
Syrup: chocolate (2 tbsp/1 fl. oz/37g)	1	0
Syrup: corn, high-fructose (1 tbsp/19g)	0	0
Syrup: malt (1 tbsp/24g)	9	2
Syrup: maple (1 tbsp/20g)	4	0
Syrup: pancake (1 tbsp/20g)	4	0

	RiskPoints ✗	LifePoints ✔
Toffee (1 piece/12g)	18	0
Tortilla chips: nacho-flavour (1 oz/28g)	18	2
Tortilla chips: plain (1 oz/28g)	18	2
Trail mix (1 oz/28g)	20	5
Truffles: mocha (standard 1 oz serving/28g)	31	1
Truffles: rum (standard 1 oz serving/28g)	41	3
Turkish delight: with nuts (standard 1 oz serving/28g)	1	0
Turkish delight: without nuts (standard 1 oz serving/28g)	0	0

Margarines, Oils & Spreads

	RiskPoints	LifePoints
Almond oil (1 tbsp/14g)	34	0
Corn oil, salad or cooking (1 tbsp/14g)	34	0
Grapeseed oil (1 tbsp/14g)	34	0
Hazelnut oil (1 tbsp/14g)	34	0
Margarine and butter blend: blend of 60% corn oil margarine and 40% butter (1 tsp/5g)	10	0
Margarine: hard, made with hydrogenated corn oil (1 tsp/4g)	9	0
Margarine: hard, made with hydrogenated soya bean oil (1 tsp/4g)	9	0
Margarine: hard, made with hydrogenated sunflower and soya bean oils (1 tsp/4g)	9	0
Margarine: low-fat (approx 40%) made with hydrogenated soya bean oil (1 tsp/4g)	4	0

	RiskPoints ✗	LifePoints ✓
Margarine: soft, made with hydrogenated or non-hydrogenated corn oil (1 tsp/4g)	9	0
Margarine: soft, made with hydrogenated or non-hydrogenated soya bean oil (1 tsp/4g)	9	0
Margarine: soft, made with hydrogenated or non-hydrogenated sunflower oil (1 tsp/4g)	9	0
Margarine: soft, made with unspecified oils (1 tsp/4g)	9	0
Olive oil: salad or cooking (1 tbsp/13.5g)	33	0
Peanut oil: salad or cooking (1 tbsp/13g)	33	0
Sesame oil: salad or cooking (1 tbsp/14g)	34	0
Soya bean oil: salad or cooking (1 tbsp/14g)	34	0
Sunflower oil: salad or cooking (1 tbsp/14g)	34	0
Vegetable shortening: made with hydrogenated soya bean and palm oils (1 tbsp/12g)	32	0
Walnut oil (1 tbsp/14g)	34	0
Wheat germ oil (1 tbsp/14g)	34	0

Herbs & Spices

Allspice: ground (1 tsp/1g)	0	0
Anise: seed (1 tsp/2g)	0	0
Basil: fresh (5 leaves/2g)	0	0
Basil: ground (1 tsp/1g)	0	0

	RiskPoints ✗	LifePoints ✔
Bay leaf: crumbled (1 tsp/1g)	0	0
Caraway: seed (1 tsp/2g)	0	0
Cardamom: ground (1 tsp/2g)	0	0
Celery: seed (1 tsp/2g)	1	0
Chervil: dried (1 tsp/1g)	0	0
Chilli: powder (1 tsp/2g)	1	1
Cinnamon: ground (1 tsp/2g)	0	1
Cloves: ground (1 tsp/2g)	1	0
Coriander: leaf, dried (1 tsp/1g)	0	0
Coriander: seed (1 tsp/1g)	0	0
Coriander: fresh (¼ cup/4g)	0	0
Cumin: seed (1 tsp/2g)	1	1
Curry: powder (1 tsp/2g)	0	0
Dill: seed (1 tsp/2g)	0	0
Dill: weed, dried (1 tsp/1g)	0	0
Dill: weed, fresh (5 sprigs/1g)	0	0
Fennel: seed (1 tsp/2g)	0	0
Fenugreek: seed (1 tsp/3g)	0	1
Garlic: powder (1 tsp/2g)	0	0
Ginger: ground (1 tsp/1g)	0	0
Mace: ground (1 tsp/1g)	1	0
Marjoram: dried (1 tsp/1g)	0	0
Mustard: seed, yellow (1 tsp/3g)	2	0
Nutmeg: ground (1 tsp/2g)	4	0
Onion: powder (1 tsp/2g)	0	0
Oregano: ground (1 tsp/1g)	0	0
Paprika (1 tsp/2g)	0	1
Parsley: dried (1 tsp/1g)	0	0
Parsley: fresh (10 sprigs/10g)	0	1

	RiskPoints ✗	LifePoints ✔
Pepper: black (1 tsp/2g)	0	0
Pepper: red or cayenne (1 tsp/1g)	0	0
Pepper: white (1 tsp/2g)	0	0
Poppy: seed (1 tsp/2g)	3	1
Rosemary: dried (1 tsp/1g)	0	0
Saffron (1 tsp/1g)	0	0
Sage: ground (1 tsp/1g)	0	0
Tarragon: ground (1 tsp/1g)	0	0
Thyme: ground (1 tsp/1g)	0	1
Turmeric: ground (1 tsp/2g)	0	0

REFERENCES

1 Harman, D., *Proc Natl Acad Sci* 1991; 88: 5360–3.
2 Harman, D. *Proc Natl Acad Sci* 1991; 88: 5360–3.
3 *Science*, 1990; 250: 634–40.
4 *Free Radicals: From Basic Science to Medicine*, Birkhauser Verlag, Basel, 1993.
5 Media statement, Alliance for Aging Research, 3 March 1994.
6 *Krause's Food Nutrition and Diet Therapy*, 8th edition, W. B. Saunders Company (US).
7 Schutz, Y., Flatt, J. P. and Jequier, E. 'Failure of Dietary Fat Intake to Promote Fat Oxidation: A Factor Favoring the Development of Obesity', *Am J Clin Nutr* 1989; 50(2): 307–14.
8 Beilin, L. J., 'Strategies and Difficulties in Dietary Intervention in Myocardial Infarction Patients', *Clin Exp Hypertens* [A] 1992; 14 (1–2): 213–221.
9 *New York Times*, 8 May 1990.
10 *New York Times*, 22 May 1991.
11 Kendall, A. et al., *Am J Clin Nutr* 1991; 53(5): 1124–9.
12 Suter, P. M. et al., *New Engl J Med* 1992; 326: 983–7.
13 *The Times*, 27 January 1988.
14 *Med Hypotheses* July 1984; 14(3).
15 *Daily Consumer News*, 30 June 1986.
16 *Acta Derm Venereol* 1984; 64(1).
17 The work of Dr Alan Ebringer, Department of Rheumatology, Middlesex Hospital, and immunologist at King's College, London.
18 Skoldstam, Lars, 'Fasting and Vegan Diet in Rheumatoid Arthritis', *Scand J Rheumatology* 1986; 15: 219–23.
19 Wayne State University College of Medicine as reported in *Better Nutrition*, March 1990; 52(3): 9(3).
20 Childers, Norman and Russo, G. M., *The Nightshades and Health*, Horticulture Publications, Somerville, New Jersey, 1973.
21 Raympiid Shatin, MD, Alfred Hospital, Melbourne, Florida, as reported in *Bestways*, September 1989; 17(9): 42(2).
22 'Yucca Plant Saponin in the Management of Arthritis', Bingham, R., Bellew, B. A. and Bellew, J. G.; *J Applied Nutr* 1975; 27: 45–50.
23 *Lancet*, 24 August 1990.
24 Various studies, including work by Professor Hans Eysenck and Dr Ronald Grossarth-Maticek, Institute of Psychiatry, London; Dr David Spiegel, Stanford University, USA.
25 *The Causes of Cancer*, R. Doll and R. Peto, Oxford Medical Publications, 1981.
26 Interview: Kenneth K. Carroll, PhD, Professor of Biochemistry, University of Western Ontario, Canada, *Redbook*, April 1989; 172(6): 96(5).

27 *Washington Post, Los Angeles Times*, 1 August 1989.

28 Michael P. Osborne, MD, of Memorial Sloan-Kettering Cancer Center, Breast Service, in conjunction with researchers at Rockefeller University, New York, and Rutgers University, New Jersey.

29 Peter Greenwald, MD; Division of Cancer Prevention and Control, National Cancer Institute.

30 Physicians' Health Study, begun 1982; Dr Charles Hennekens, Harvard Medical School and Brigham & Women's Hospital, Boston National Cancer Institute, Cancer Research Laboratory, Bethesda, Maryland, USA; Regina Ziegler, PhD, Environmental Epidemiology Department.

31 'Can Vitamins Help Prevent Cancer?', *Consumer Reports*, May 1983; 48(5): 243–5.

32 *Redbook*, April 1989; 172(6): 96(5).

33 'Good Diet Curbs Cancer Risk', *The Independent*, 3 October 1989.

34 Gerhard Schrauzer, PhD, of the University of California, cited in *Better Nutrition*, November 1989; 51(11): 14(2).

35 *Redbook*, April 1989; 172(6): 96(5).

36 'Advances in the Role of Minerals in Immunology', Spallholz, J. E., Stewart, J. R., Center for Food and Nutrition, Texas Tech University, Lubbock 79409. *Biol Trace Elem Res Mar* 1989; 19(3): 129–51.

37 *Archives of Environmental Health*, September/October 1976.

38 Knekt, Paul, et al., 'Selenium Deficiency and Increased Risk of Lung Cancer', abstract of a paper read at the Fourth International Symposium on Selenium in Biology and Medicine, Tübingen, Germany, July 1988.

39 Reinhold, U., et al.,'Selenium Deficiency and Lethal Skin Cancer', abstract of a paper read at the Fourth International Symposium on Selenium in Biology and Medicine, Tübingen, Germany, July 1988.

40 *Nutrition Almanac*, Nutrition Search, Inc., McGraw-Hill Company.

41 American Cancer Society, nutritional guidelines, *Health*, June 1984; 16:9 (1).

42 *Probiotics*, Leon Chaitow, ND, DO, and Tatasha Trenev, Thorsons, 1990.

43 'The Consumption of Seaweed as a Protective Factor in the Etiology of Breast Cancer', J. Teas, *Med Hypotheses* 1981; 7(5): 601–13.

44 'Can Vitamins Help Cancer?', *Consumer Reports*, May 1983; 48(5): 243–5.

45 'Effects of an Oats Fibre Tablet and Wheat Bran in Healthy Volunteers', Vorster, H. H., Lotter, A. P. and Odendaal, I. S., *S. Afr Med J*, 29 March 1986.

46 'Hypocholesterolemic Effects of Oat-bran or Bean Intake for Hyper-cholesterolemic Men', Anderson, J. W., Story, L., Sieling, B., Chen, W. J., Petro, M. S. and Story, J., *American Journal of Clinical Nutrition*, December 1984.

47 Delthia Ricks, UPI, 17 March 1988.

48 'Dietary Fiber Content of Selected Foods', Anderson, J. W. and Bridges, S. R., *American Journal of Clinical Nutrition*, March 1988.

49 'Hypocholesterolemic Effects of Oat and Bean Products', Anderson,

J. W. and Gustafson, *American Journal of Clinical Nutrition*, September 1988.

50 *The Times*, 8 February 1988.

51 ' "Yuppie Flu" Turns Out to Be Real', *Los Angeles Times*, 24 January 1991.

52 *Washington Post*, 27 November 1990.

53 *Patient Care*, 15 November 1987; 21(18): 79(4).

54 *Better Nutrition for Today's Living*, May 1990; 52–5: 20(4).

55 *Better Nutrition for Today's Living*, May 1990; 52–5: 20(4).

56 UPI, 19 December 1990.

57 *Independent*, 30 April 1991.

58 *The Atlantic*, Sept 1987, 260: 56(16).

59 *Holistic Medicine*, March–April 1990: 8(2).

60 *Chronic Fatigue Syndrome: The Hidden Epidemic*, Jesse Stoff and Charles Pellegrino, Random House, 1988.

61 UPI, 1 March 1990.

62 'Vitamin C as a Preventive Medicine Against Common Colds in Children', Ludvigsson, J., Hansson, L. O. and Tibbling, G., *Scand J Infect Dis* 1977; 9(2): 91–8.

63 'Large Scale Studies with Vitamin C', Anderson, T. W., *Acta Vitaminol Enzymol* 1977; 31(1–5): 43–50.

64 'Reduction in Duration of Common Colds by Zinc Gluconate Lozenges in a Double-Blind Study', Eby, G. A., Davis, D. R. and Halcomb, W. W., *Antimicrob Agents Chemother*, January 1984; 25(1): 20–4.

65 'Role of Sugars in Human Neutrophilic Phagocytosis', Sanchez, A., Reeser, J. L., Lau, H. S., Yahiku, P. Y., Willard, R. E., McMillan, P. J., Cho, S. Y., Magie, A. R. and Register, U. D., *Am J Clin Nutr*, November 1973; 26(11): 1180–4.

66 National Advisory Committee on Nutrition Education, *Proposals for Nutritional Guidelines for Health Education in Britain*, The Health Education Council, September 1983.

67 *Introducing Diabetes*, British Diabetic Association.

68 *Diabetes in the United Kingdom, 1988*, British Diabetic Association.

69 *Diabetes in the United Kingdom, 1988*, British Diabetic Association.

70 'Preventing Insulin Dependent Diabetes Mellitus: the Environmental Challenge', Diabetes Epidemiology Research International, *British Medical Journal* (Clinical Research), 22 August 1987; 295(6596): 479–81.

71 'Nutritional Recommendations and Principles for Individuals With Diabetes Mellitus: 1986', *American Diabetes Association: Diabetes Care*, January–February 1987; 10(1).

72 'Does a Vegetarian Diet Reduce the Occurrence of Diabetes?', Snowdon, David A. and Phillips, Roland L., *American Journal of Public Health*, May 1985; 75(5).

73 'Does a Vegetarian Diet Reduce the Occurrence of Diabetes?', Snowdon, David A. and Phillips, Roland L., *American Journal of Public Health*, May 1985; 75(5).

74 'Coffee Consumption as Trigger for Insulin Dependent Diabetes Mellitus in Childhood', Tuomilehto, J., et al., Department of Epidemiology, National Public Health Institute, Helsinki, Finland, *British Medical Journal*, 10 March 1990; 300(6725): 642–3.

75 [Dermatomycoses and an antifungal diet] 'Haurmykosen und Antipilz-diat', Putzier, E., *Wien Med Wochenschr* (Austria), 31 August 1989; 139(15–16); 379–80.

76 Sir James Black, quoted in *The Independent*, 22 October 1988.

77 Sir James Black, quoted in *The Independent*, 22 October 1988; John J. Voorhees, MD, Department of Dermatology, University of Michigan Medical School, Ann Arbor, Michigan, USA, reported in *Archives of Dermatology* and *Better Nutrition for Today's Living*, June 1990; 52(6): 22–3.

78 Donald O. Rudin, MD, *The Omega-3 Phenomenon* and *Better Nutrition for Today's Living*, June 1990; 52(6): 22–3.

79 *Better Nutrition for Today's Living*, June 1990; 52(6): 22–3.

80 Fry, L., et al., 'The Mechanism of Folate Deficiency in Psoriasis', *British Journal of Dermatology* 1971; 84: 539–44.

81 'Influence of Maternal Diet During Lactation and Use of Formula Feeds on Development of Atopic Eczema in High Risk Infants', Chandra Ranjit Kumar, Puri, Shakuntla and Hamed, Azza, *British Medical Journal*, 22 July 1989; 298(6693); 228(3).

82 'A Fasting and Vegetarian Diet Treatment Trial on Chronic Inflammatory Disorders'. Lithell, H., et al., *Acta Derm Venereol* (Stockh) 1983; 63(5): 397–403.

83 Dr Kari Poilolainen, et al., National Public Health Institute, Helsinki, as reported in the *BMJ* and *The Independent*, 23 March 1990.

84 *British Medical Journal*, July 1985.

85 *Los Angeles Times*, 18 July 1989.

86 *HeartCorps*, December 1989; 2(3): 67(4).

87 *HeartCorps*, December 1989; 2(3): 67(4).

88 'Relation of Moderate Alcohol Consumption and Risk of Systemic Hypertension in Women', Witteman, Jacqueline C. M., et al., *American Journal of Cardiology*, 1 March 1990, 65(9): 633(5).

89 *Journal of the American Medical Association*, 11 April 1990.

90 'A Vegan Regimen with Reduced Medication in the Treatment of Hypertension', Lindahl, O., et al., *Br J Nutr*, July 1984; 52(1): 11–20.

91 'Randomised Blind Controlled Trial of a High Fibre, Low Fat and Low Sodium Dietary Regimen in Mild Essential Hypertension', Dodson, et al., *J Hum Hypertens*, June 1989; 3(3): 197–202.

92 'Consumption of Olive Oil, Butter, and Vegetable Oils and Coronary Heart Disease Risk Factors', Trevisan, et al., *Journal of the American Medical Association*, 2 February 1990; 263(5): 688(5).

93 'Nutritional Aspects of Hypertension', Seedat, Y. K., *S Afr Med J* (South Africa), 18 February 1989; 75(4): 175–7.

94 *Better Nutrition*, July 1990; 52(7):14(2).

95 'Serum Calcium and Salt Restriction in the Diet of Patients with Essential

Arterial Hypertension', Uza, G. and Vlaicu, R., et al., *Med Interne*, April–June 1989; 27(2): 93–7.

96 *Medical World News*, 26 February 1990; 31(4): 22(2).

97 *FDA Consumer*, February 1989; 23(1): 10(5).

98 *Journal of the American Medical Association*, 21 October 1988.

99 'Controlled Trial of Oligoantigenic Treatment in the Hyperkinetic Syndrome', Egger, J., Carter, C. M., Graham, P. J., Gumley, D. and Soothill, J. F., *Lancet*, 9 March 1985; 1(8428): 540–5.

100 'The Northern California Diet-Behavior Program: an Empirical Examination of 3,000 Incarcerated Juveniles in Stanislaus County Juvenile Hall', Schoenthaler, Stephen J., *International Journal of Biosocial Research* 1983; 5(2): 99–106.

101 'Types of Offenses which can be Reduced in an Institutional Setting Using Nutritional Intervention: a Preliminary Empirical Evaluation', Schoenthaler, Stephen J. and Doraz, Walter E., *International Journal for Biosocial Research* 1983; 4(2): 74–84.

102 'Role of Sugars in Human Neutrophilic Phagocytosis', Sanchez, A., et al., *Am J Clin Nutr*, November 1973; 26(11): 1180–4.

103 Alkohol og infeksjoner. Morland, B., Morland, H., Norges allmennvitenskapelige forskningsr. ANG. ad, Oslo. Tidsskr Nor Laegeforen, 1990; 110(4): 490–3. 'Neutrophil elastase activity and superoxide production are diminished in neutrophils of alcoholics', Sachs, C. W., Christensen, R. H., Pratt, P. C., Lynn, W. S., Department of Pathology, Duke University School of Medicine, Durham, North Carolina, *Am Rev Respir Dis*, May 1990; 141(5 Pt 1); 1249–55.

104 'Human Neutrophils are Not Severely Injured in Conditions Mimicking Social Drinking', Corberand, J. X., Laharrague, P. F. and Fillola, G., Central Laboratory of Haematology, CHU Rangueil, Toulouse, France, *Alcohol Clin Exp Res*, August 1989; 13(4): 542–6.

105 'Role of Sugars in Human Neutrophilic Phagocytosis', Sanchez, A., et al., *Am J Clin Nutr*, November 1973; 26(11):1180–4.

106 'Role of Life-style and Dietary Habits in Risk of Cancer among Seventh-Day Adventists', Roland L. Phillips, *Cancer Research*, November 1975; 35:3513–22.

107 'Vitamin B6 Deficiency and Carcinogenesis', Reynolds, R. D., US Department of Agriculture, Beltsville Human Nutrition Research Center, Maryland. *Adv Exp Med Biol*, 1986; 206:339–47.

108 'Suppression of Tumor Growth and Enhancement of Immune Status with High Levels of Dietary Vitamin B6 in BALB/c Mice', Gridley, D. S., Stickney, D. R., Nutter, R. L., Slater, J. M. and Shultz, T. D. *J Natl Cancer Inst*, May 1987; 78(5): 951–9.

109 'Vitamin B6 Revisited. Evidence of Subclinical Deficiencies in Various Segments of the Population and Possible Consequences Thereof', Serfontein, W. J., De Villiers, L. S., Ubbink, J. and Pitout, M. J., *S Afr Med J*, 22 September 1984; 66(12): 437–41.

110 'Pyridoxine Supplementation: Effect on Lymphocyte Responses in

Elderly Persons', Talbott, M. C., Miller, L. T. and Kerkvliet, N. I., Department of Foods and Nutrition, Oregon State University, Corvallis, *Am J Clin Nutr*, October 1987; 46(4): 659–64.

111 American Hospital Formulary Service, American Society of Hospital Pharmacists, 1990.

112 'Vitamin E and Immune Functions', Bendich, A., Clinical Nutrition, Hoffmann La Roche Inc., Nutley, New Jersey, *Basic Life Sci* 1988; 49:615–20.

113 'Vitamin E and Immune Functions', Bendich, A., Clinical Nutrition, Hoffmann La Roche Inc., Nutley, New Jersey, *Basic Life Sci* 1988; 49: 615–20.

114 *Basic Life Science* 1988; 49: 615–20.

115 Berger, Stuart, MD, 'Learning More About Viruses', *New York Post*, 9 May 1989.

116 'The Effect of Ascorbic Acid Deficiency on Leukocyte Phagocytosis and Killing of Actinomyces Viscosus', Goldschmidt, M. et al., *Int J Vitam Nutr Res*, 1988; 58(3): 326–34.

117 *Better Nutrition*, April 1989; 51(4): 16(3).

118 'Immunostimulatory Effects of Beta-Carotene on T-cell Activation Markers and NK Cells in HIV Infected Patients', Watson, R. R., et al., *Int Conf AIDS*, 4–9 June 1989; 5: 663.

119 'Nutrition and Immune Responses', Chandra, R. K., *Can J Physiol Pharmacol*, March 1983; 61(3): 290–4.

120 *Nutrition Reports International*, 1988; 17: 157–63.

121 *Better Nutrition*, January 1989; 51: 10(4).

122 Drs John Martin, Colorado State University, and Julian E. Spallholz, Long Beach, California Veterans Administration Hospital, cited in *Better Nutrition*, November 1989; 51(11): 14(2).

123 Gerhard Schrauzer, PhD, of the University of California, cited in *Better Nutrition*, November 1989; 51(11): 14(2).

124 *Redbook*, April 1989; 172(6): 96(5).

125 'Macrophage Activation and Induction of Macrophage Cytotoxicity by Purified Polysaccharide Fractions from the Plant Echinaceae Purpurea', Stimpel, M. et al., *Infection Immunity* 1984; 46: 845–9.

126 *Potter's New Cyclopedia of Botanical Drugs and Preparations*, R. C. Wren, C. W. Daniel Company Ltd, 1982.

127 Kumazawa, Y., et al., 'Activation of Peritoneal Macrophages by Berinedtype Alkaloids in Terms of Induction of Cytostatic Activity', *Int J Immunopharmac* 1984; 6: 587–92.

128 Abe, N., et al., 'Interferon Induction by Glycyrrhiz and Glycyrrhetinic Acid in Mice', *Microbial Immunol*, 1982; 26: 535–9.

129 Pompeii, R., et al., 'Antiviral Activity of Glycyrrhizic Acid', *Experentia* 1980; 36: 304–5.

130 Mitscher, L., et al., 'Antimicrobial Agents from Higher Plants. Antimicrobial Isoflavonoids from Glycyrrhiza Glabra L. var typica', *J. Nat. Products*, 1980; 43: 259–69.

131 *Potter's New Cyclopedia of Botanical Drugs and Preparations*, R. C. Wren, C. W. Daniel Company Ltd, 1982.

132 *Today's Living*, September 1989; 20(9): 5(6).

133 Cited in *Better Nutrition*, January 1989; 51(1): 10(4).

134 'Garlic as an Antimicrobial and Immune Modulator in AIDS', Abdullah, T., Kirkpatrick, D. V., Williams, L. and Carter, J., Akbar Research Foundation, Panama City, Florida, USA, *Int Conf AIDS*, 4–9 June 1989; 5: 466.

135 'Green Tea Cuts Cancerous Growths', *New Scientist*, 12 September 1987.

136 'Milk Intolerance in Children with Persistent Sleeplessness: a Prospective Double-blind Crossover Evaluation', Kahn, A., et al., Pediatric Sleep Unit, University Children's Hospital, Free University of Brussels, Belgium; *Pediatrics*, October 1989; 84(4): 596–603. 'Sleep Characteristics in Milk-intolerant Infants', Kahn, A., et al., *Sleep* (US), June 1988; 11(3): 291–7. 'Difficulty in Initiating and Maintaining Sleep Associated with Cow's Milk Allergy in Infants', Kahn, A., et al., *Sleep* (US), April 1987; 10(2): 116–21.

137 'Is Migraine Food Allergy? A Double-blind Controlled Trial of Oligoantigenic Diet Treatment', Egger, J., Carter, C. M., Wilson, J., Turner, M. W. and Soothill, J. F., *Lancet*, 15 October 1983; 2 (8355): 865–9.

138 *Living*, April 1990; 21(4): 14(3).

139 'Efficacy of Feverfew as Prophylactic Treatment of Migraine', Johnson, E. S., Kadam, N. P., Hylands, D. M. and Hylands, P. J., *Br Med J Clin Res*, 31 August 1985; 291(6495): 569–73.

140 'Randomised Double-blind Placebo-controlled Trial of Feverfew in Migraine Prevention', Murphy, J. J., Heptinstall, S. and Mitchell, J. R., Department of Medicine, University Hospital, Nottingham, *Lancet*, 23 July 1988; 2(8604): 189–92.

141 Wang, J. P., et al., 'Antiplatelet Effect of Capsaicin', *Thrombosis Research*, 1984: 497–507.

142 Dr John McDougall, *Vegetarian Times*, June 1989; 142: 60(3).

143 *American Journal of Medicine*, 1950; 220: 421.

144 'Multiple Sclerosis: Twenty Years on Low Fat Diet'. Swank, R. L., *Arch. Neurol*, November 1970; 23(5): 460–74.

145 *The Multiple Sclerosis Diet Book*, Swank, R. L. and Pullen, M. H., Doubleday, Garden City, New York, 1977.

146 *The Edell Health Letter*, May 1989; 8(5): 6(1).

147 'Low-fat Diet May Cut Deaths from MS', Celia Hall, *Independent*, 6 July 1990.

148 'Effect of Low Saturated Fat Diet in Early and Late Cases of Multiple Sclerosis', Swank, Roy Laver; Dugan, Barbara Brewer, *Lancet*, 7 July 1990; 336(8706): 37(3).

149 *Lancet*, 7 July 1990; 336(8706): 25(2).

150 Dr John McDougall, *Vegetarian Times*, June 1989; 142: 60(3).

151 Newsletter of the National Osteoporosis Society no. 1.

152 National Osteoporosis Society leaflet no. 2.

153 *Independent*, 23 October 1990.

154 John Studd, Consultant Gynaecologist, King's College & Dulwich Hospitals, Vice-Chairman of the National Osteoporosis Society.

155 *The Independent*, 23 October 1990.

156 'Postmenopausal Osteoporosis: Its Clinical Features', Albright, F., Smith, P. H. and Richardson, A. M., *JAMA* 1941; 116: 2465–74.

157 'Estrogen Replacement Therapy for the Prevention of Osteoporosis', Lufkin, Edward G. and Ory, Steven J., *American Family Physician*, September 1989; 40(3): 205(7).

158 Mack, T. M., Pike, M. C., Henderson, B. E., et al., 'Estrogens and Endometrial Cancer in a Retirement Community', *N Engl J Med* 1976; 294: 1262–7.

159 'A Risk-benefit Assessment of Estrogen Therapy in Postmenopausal Women', Cust, M. P., Gangar, K. F., Hillard, T. C. and Whitehead, M. I., Academic Department of Obstetrics and Gynaecology, King's College School of Medicine and Dentistry, London, England, *Drug Saf*, September–October 1990; 5 (5): 345–58.

160 'Hormone-replacement Therapy and the Risk of Breast Cancer', Hulka, B. S., Department of Epidemiology, University of North Carolina, Chapel Hill, *CA*, September–October 1990; 40(5): 289–96.

161 'Estrogen Replacement Therapy for the Prevention of Osteoporosis', Lufkin, Edward G. and Ory, Steven J., *American Family Physician*, September 1989; 40(3): 205(7).

162 'Effects of Nitrogen Phosphorus, and Caffeine on Calcium Balance in Women', Heaney, R. P. and Recker, R. R., *J Lab Clin Med*, January 1982; 99(1): 46–55.

163 *What Everyone Needs to Know about Osteoporosis*, The National Osteoporosis Society.

164 'Research Advances in Osteoporosis', Conference by the National Osteoporosis Foundation, the National Institutes of Health, and the American Society of Bone and Mineral Research, Arlington, Virginia, USA, February 1990.

165 'Osteoporosis, Calcium Requirement, and Factors Causing Calcium Loss', Spencer, H. and Kramer, L., *Clin Geriatr Med*, May 1987; 3(2): 389–402.

166 'Vegetarian Lifestyle and Bone Mineral Density', Marsh, A. G., Sanchez, T. V., Michelsen, O., Chaffee, F. L. and Fagal, S. M., Department of Home Economics, Andrews University, Berrien Springs, Michigan, *Am J Clin Nutr*, September 1988; 48 (3 Suppl): 837–41.

167 'Relationship of Animal Protein-rich Diet to Kidney Stone Formation and Calcium Metabolism', Breslau, N. A., Brinkley, L., Hill, K. D. and Pak, C. Y., Center in Mineral Metabolism and Clinical Research, Department of Internal Medicine, Dallas, Texas, *J Clin Endocrinol Metab*, January 1988; 66(1): 140–6.

168 'Effect of Dietary Boron on Mineral, Estrogen, and Testosterone Metabolism in Postmenopausal Women', Nielsen, F. H., Hunt, C. D., Mullen,

L. M. and Hunt, J. R., United States Department of Agriculture, Grand Forks Human Nutrition Research Center, North Dakota, *FASEB J*, November 1987; 1(5): 394–7.

169 'Osteoporosis Strategies for Prevention', White, J. E., Family Nurse Practitioner Program, University of Pittsburgh School of Nursing, *Nurse Pract*, 1986; 11(9): 36–46, 50.

170 *Gut* 1989; 30: 1201–5.

171 *Nutrition Health Review*, Fall 1989; 52: 4(1).

172 *Nutrition Health Review*, Fall 1989; 52: 4(1).

INDEX

Page numbers in *italic* refer either to Top Ten foods (pages 114–18) or to Food Counter scores (pages 191–325). A list of named recipes is found under 'recipes'.